YOU
ARE NOT
ALONE:

Compulsive Hair Pulling
"The Enemy Within"

D1563995

Cheryn Salazar

ROPHE PRESS
Sacramento, Californa

3rd Edition

DEDICATION

To my husband, Michael, whom I love and appreciate with all of my heart. You are my best friend and I thank you for the sensitivity and respect that you have given me in our marriage.

To my children Jessica, Alyson, Mikaela and Michael II, who have given their loving support and patience to me in my writing of this book. I couldn't have asked for more wonderful children. I love and am truly grateful for each of you.

To Rene Strasser, who is my surrogate "sister" and my dearest friend. You have been a vital person in my life. I have been truly blessed with your friendship. I love you very much.

To Christina Pearson, who is my dear friend, confidant and sounding board. You have stood by me through many experiences in my life and you have given me a safe place to learn and grow. Thank you for your friendship.

To Marcia Zina Mager, who offered her own experience and expertise, as an author, to me during the beginning stages of writing my book. Thank you for your help.

And to my parents, Keith and Cynthia Larkin, who have been an example to me of people who care about other people. Thank you for your love and support. Your example of caring and generosity has impacted my life and that of many others. It is such an honor to have you as my parents.

iv

TABLE OF CONTENTS

INTRODUCTION 1

Chapter 1 9
WHAT IS TRICHOTILLOMANIA?

Chapter 2 15
MY STORY

Chapter 3 49
ISOLATION & DEPRESSION

Chapter 4 65
IDENTIFYING SHAME, ANXIETIES
& EMOTIONS

Chapter 5 89
CODEPENDENCY &
POSITIVE AFFIRMATIONS

Chapter 6 113
TRIGGERS FOR PULLING/
RELAXATION TECHNIQUES

Chapter 7 127
A PARENT'S STORY

Chapter 8 137
A CHILD'S STORY

Chapter 9 149
A MATE'S STORY

Chapter 10 165
RECOVERY

Chapter 11 199
JOURNAL ENTRIES & POETRY CLIPS

Chapter 12 221
TRICHOTILLOMANIA
LEARNING CENTER (TLC)

Chapter 13 225
CONCLUSION

SUGGESTED READING
AUDIO/VISUAL AIDS & PRODUCTS 231

"OUR POEM"

I am tired from the many years and tears

This affliction has taken me through—not around

There have been no shortcuts, no paved roads

But a pathway that's been taken by many

That have been without human help

Without given direction

Now with binding faith in a sister/brotherhood

We now see we have unknowingly traveled
hand in hand

We've cried similar tears in isolation

Yet the tears gathered and kept by a gentle hand

And placed in a lake

To later immerse all who have contributed

With arms of familiarity

Embracing around each other's hearts

We will cry no more of pain

But of the joys of finding the lake

Finding each other

©1990 Cheryn Salazar

INTRODUCTION

INTRODUCTION

This is my story, a mixture of my journals, poems, and topics that reach deep into my soul. I know that I am not alone now, and I want you to know that you are not alone. My desire is to reach out to the many millions, yes that's right, millions of men, women and children who still think they are the only ones. I want to share my story and my steps of hope, hair pulling, and a deeper recovery than I ever imagined there could be.

Today I embrace my Trichotillomania with gratefulness because it has forced me to grow from the inside out. I have come to a knowledge of myself that I truly believe would have never come without the depth of pain and soul searching that Trich has put me through.

Do you want to have your hair? I mean, how hard are you willing to work to get it? This is no easy road. With the support from other pullers, and perhaps a therapist, and a willingness to look deep within yourself, I believe with all my heart and soul that you can overcome the compulsion to pull. Diffusing the issues, emotions, and physical impulses that precede and trigger pulling episodes and someday having hair is possible.

In 1984 I experienced a great relief after reading an Ann Landers article, finding out that I wasn't alone. It was to be the catalyst for a new beginning in my life. When I read a letter about another person with

Trichotillomania, there was a connection deep in my spirit.

I remember opening up the newspaper over at some relative's house and reading Ann's column from a mother of a daughter who pulled out her lashes. I was stunned and breathless. The impact was like lightning striking a forbidden area of hurt and isolation inside my soul. I quickly shut the paper and sat there with many emotions spinning around in my mind. "I am not alone," I silently screamed.

My prayer and desire is that we can be the new generation that no longer has to hide and doesn't have to suffer in isolation and depression, with the feelings of abnormalcy that Trichotillomania brings. I hope that you can be helped emotionally as well as physically through the words of this book. I wish there had been such a book available for me to read so that I could have felt a deliverance from the isolation I've experienced, a source of help to overcome the repercussions we experience with Trichotillomania. That is actually what prompted the writing of this book.

However, as the years have gone by in my writing the chapters of this book, I have realized that there is much more needed than just identification with others. The last part of this introduction gives an explanation that I hope will help make Trichotillomania comprehensible to you. I believe understanding is essential in alleviating the shame that binds us, freeing us to be able to grow and become whole. I know that it helped me immensely to find out there was a medical term and definition for what I have experienced since 1972. It helps us all to know that we are neither "weird" nor "crazy."

I also write about ways to diffuse the behaviors that often precipitate pulling episodes, the actual benefits I have gained, and other stories and anecdotes.

We are all pioneers, crossing new land on roads that have not been previously paved for us. Be courageous and go forth, being willing to break through the obstacles that have so far kept us all bound. In doing so, you will be helping not only yourself, but the future generations who will encounter Trichotillomania. They already have the blessing of knowing that they are not alone. What a wonderful gift they have already received! This is just the beginning for them . . . for all of us.

I have written this book with tears and deep emotion for all of you, all of us, with Trichotillomania. I wish I could embrace each one of you. I think you understand what I mean. There is an understanding that we all share, isn't there? I am grateful for every single person I have met who shares my experience. I liken it to being long lost twins who may have never met, but we know each other. We know each other's pain.

This book will cover several periods and years of my life, sharing the experiences which I hope will speak to and be identified with by other sufferers of Trichotillomania. I surely do not use the word "suffering" lightly. We know suffering. I believe we suffer until we can face and overcome our underlying issues that give us our impulse to pull.

Christina Pearson describes Trichotillomania as a **"neuro-emotive"** disorder. She sees it as "a neural agitation (from what, she is not sure; perhaps problems in the neurotransmitter systems). This neural agitation creates an emotional chemistry that is displaced into a physiological behavior mechanism instead of an emotional expression."

I believe we can reduce some contributing neurological aggravators by using methods which will diffuse the anxiety "buttons" that often trigger pulling sprees. One method is by relaxing using breathing techniques. Another way is by reducing or eliminating caffeine and sugar.

I believe the emotive (emotional) aspect is approachable and correctable through the process of learning what precedes our pulling episodes. We must become aware of and identify our feelings. I liken it to the peeling of an onion, one layer at a time. (We all know what happens when we peel an onion. Tears. Lots of tears.)

As we "peel and remove the layers" of dysfunctional behaviors, by learning the whys and hows of them, we are then able to learn a new way to live. Then we can let go of the old destructive behaviors and begin to heal and change from the inside out, with pulling often being the last to be alleviated. (The twelve steps used in my recovery programs have been very beneficial in my learning a new way to live.) Our outlook on life, people and ourselves will become less stressful if we are willing to walk this road.

I don't know if we can ever completely stop pulling, but I do know from my own experience that my pulling has been drastically reduced. The duration of time between pulling episodes has lengthened. If the "aggravator buttons" are removed, recovery happens. It most likely will be a slow process, but well worth the wait. I believe the longer you have pulled, the longer time it will take to recover. So be patient. There are no quick answers.

I believe that once we put the key of willingness in the door, the door opens on its own, with its own perfect timing. I have found the process to be quite gentle. The outcome is peace and freedom. Come. Let us walk this road hand in hand. You are not alone anymore.

1

WHAT IS TRICHOTILLOMANIA?

Christina Pearson, founder and Executive Director of the Trichotillomania Learning Center, wrote up an easy-to-comprehend pamphlet to help inform anyone interested in learning about this disorder. She has allowed me to reprint her pamphlet in this chapter.

Trichotillomania is an anxiety disorder that manifests itself in the compulsive urge to pull one's hair, resulting in noticeable hair loss. Currently defined in medical literature as an impulse control disorder, the condition has come to light in recent years. This is the result of media attention on Obsessive-Compulsive Disorder. There are distinct differences in these conditions, but there is enough of an overlap that compulsive hair pulling is commonly included in what are called "Obsessive-Compulsive Spectrum Disorders." These include a variety of conditions that seem related to OCD, but do not meet actual OCD diagnostic criterion.

The term "Trichotillomania" is derived from the Greek words for hair (thrix), to pull out (tillein), and insanity, or frenzy (mania). It was coined in 1889 by a French dermatologist named Hallepeau for describing the case of a young man.

Many people are affected by this disorder. Sufferers, who range in all ages, but many of whom are children under the age of ten, experience profound shame, hopelessness, depression and embarrassment that can impact every aspect of their lives. There are some that have worn wigs, hair pieces and false eyelashes for as long as they can remember. Children who have never ridden on a roller coaster for fear of the wind. People who cannot swim, bike, run, dance, or be in a relationship. They fear the exposure of their hidden secret. Children who refuse to go to school because of the ridicule they experience from other classmates. Parents who cannot provide help or compassion because they do not understand the nature of the disorder, and many doctors who fail to diagnose the condition because they have not been trained to do so.

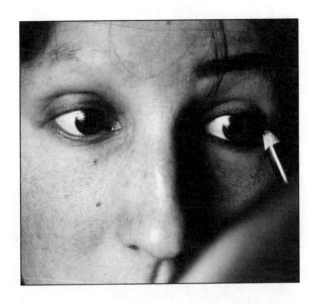

2

MY STORY

This book is for you, as well as for me. It has been very cathartic in my life, for it has been like a big journal. I hope that you will benefit from it and be able to identify a part of you with me, that you perhaps have never before experienced. Thank you for letting me share a part of my life with you.

For several years now I have been looking back into my childhood, hoping to find answers to many of my questions. I have found answers to most of my questions, but one of my biggest unanswered questions has been, "Why do I pull out my eyelashes, eyebrows and other body hair?"

I do not have all the answers, just as doctors are still unclear about all aspects of it. But I believe I have developed a pretty good idea of several factors in my life that explain the existence of my Trichotillomania.

To begin with, there are a few members in my family tree, that I am aware of, who have experienced Trichotillomania or an obsessive compulsive behavior in varying manifestations and degrees. One relative mildly pulled her eyelashes, another compulsively cut her hair, and another relative compulsively washed his hands. Unfortunately, my family was very distant from all our relatives, so I know of no others who might also have had Trichotillomania.

Now I'll tell you my story . . .

I know that I was a typical kid in most ways, but deep inside I felt like I wasn't as accepted as everyone else. Physical abilities and a good attitude in my personality didn't come easy to me, and I held the impression that everyone else was mostly happy and secure with themselves. I definitely felt a loneliness inside.

I was raised in an extremely wealthy family and was physically provided for very well. My parents loved me very much. They both were very beautiful, self-disciplined and successful people. They seemed to be able to accomplish anything they set their minds to.

I felt I was always the "difficult" child. I definitely felt my parents' frustration with me, for I was moody and combative. I always felt I didn't quite measure up to them.

I was the youngest of three children, with a sister and a brother. My sister was almost three years older. She was an honor student in school, always getting straight A's, and she was an active tomboy and accomplished equestrian. Later in high school she was very popular with the boys and seemed to get along well with everybody. (The most popular boys from three local high schools pursued her! And not for the reasons you're probably thinking!) My sister and I were not particularly close. We played together as kids, but

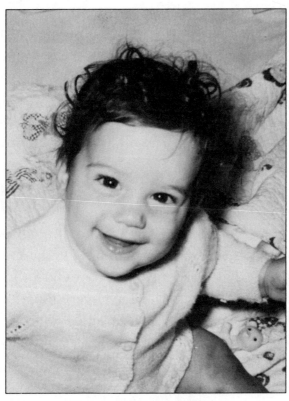

Cheryn: 10 months old

she preferred her other friends' company as we grew older.

My brother is seven years older and unfortunately we were too far apart in age to be very close. I knew that he also was difficult in his adolescent years, but by the time he moved out, I was the "teen" and I now filled the "difficult child" spot.

My parents loved and cared for me, doing their best to raise me, but they were unable to provide the emotional communication that I now recognize I desperately needed.

Back in my parents' generation, they lived what they learned as children, and I believe my parents didn't have much of an emotional relationship with their parents as I now experience with my parents. I know as a child, growing up, they loved me. They were endearing to me with affection and they gave me everything I needed and could just about have ever wanted. They certainly did their best in the roles of parenting that they could.

My dad was very successful financially and my mother was very successful in the home. He became a self-made millionaire by his early forties and she always kept the inside as well as the outside of our home looking immaculate. She always had me looking nice. There was no physical or sexual abuse or anything like that. What I needed was contact on an emotional level that they did not know how to give me and I didn't even know I needed. (Today children in our society are thought of very differently than they were thirty years ago. Communication is also a skill that was not emphasized between parent and child as it is today.)

I needed to learn what life and people were about. As an adult I realized that my parents couldn't give me what they didn't possess themselves. My parents gave everything they had and I respect them for that today and I honor and love them. But I needed my parents to be a type of guide to help me through life, like a gymnast has a "spotter" to help them as they learn their routines.

As I mentioned before, I had a very challenging and difficult personality. I would test just about every boundary they set for me and I managed to manipulate them most times with my persistent whining. I remember feeling very insecure inside. I now recognize why. I didn't have the boundaries I needed and unknowingly wanted as a child.

I was always hungering for attention. I faked injuries to get attention emotionally and physically, and to feel important. I wanted to feel nurtured. Unfortunately, I have several severe examples of this.

I pretended I needed glasses when I was in fifth grade. In my grammar school there was an annual hearing and vision test for all students. The day of my vision test I purposely failed the test and my mom took me to an eye doctor. I pretended to be unable able to see well and was fitted for glasses. That evening I sincerely admitted tearfully that I had lied. My parents forgave me and my mom made another appointment to have my eyes tested so that she could see how they really were. I lied again! I did this time and time again with hearing appointments, too.

I was always wanting attention by feigning injury. One time when I was at Deer Valley Camp (which my parents owned), I slipped on soap and fell in the shower. I was startled for a second and then I made it into a major thing. I was taken to the hospital where they x-rayed me and gave me a neck brace.

The next year at the same camp there was an automobile accident. Some people fell off a flat-bed trailer which was being towed by a jeep. The jeep's brakes went out, and the driver saw a cliff on one side and a mountain on the other side. She ran the jeep and the trailer up the hill. As the jeep and the wagon jackknifed, some kids fell off the back end. When the trailer rolled backwards down the hill it ran over one boy's leg with a tire and the tail pipe went up the leg of another boy. And then there was me. I didn't fall off the trailer, I just bounced around a little. Once the commotion was over, I started complaining that my leg hurt, too. I went to the hospital and was put in a

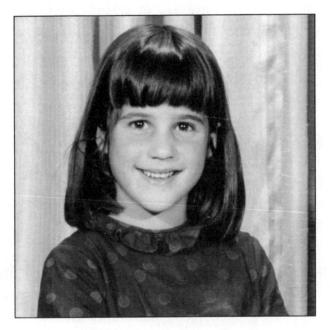

Cheryn: Second Grade

wheelchair with a full ace bandage on my leg. Of course they could find no injury, but because of the way I complained they had to treat my injury as a sprain.

I didn't know how to ask and receive attention appropriately. Back then I had no clue as to why I would do these things. I just knew that I felt bad inside for doing these "bad" things.

I didn't feel peaceful inside myself in other ways as well. I had a high level of anxiety, and school was always a struggle for me. I had a difficult time focusing my attention. (Today I believe the problem was, at least partially, caused by Attention Deficit Disorder (ADD) which was not known about back then as it is now.) I just figured I was stupid and incapable to do things the "smarter" kids could do.

Boys were of big interest to me, because their attention toward me made me feel that I had some value. I always felt a need to be liked, and since girlfriend relationships were virtually unknown to me, boys' attention met this need.

From five years old and on I had boyfriends. I don't think I was ever without a boyfriend, or at least not looking for one. I was called "boy crazy." I know I was loved by my parents, but there was something inside me that needed more. I didn't have love for myself, so I tried to create other ways to make myself feel loved. This caused a very troublesome life for me.

In school I felt a huge sense of unacceptance. There were many groups of people who were friends and it bothered me deeply that I never belonged to any such group. Today as I observe my own two teenage daughters' friendships with their best friends, I recognize that they possess an emotional quality and depth between them. They can share their innermost secrets with each other.

I know that I missed out on that in my own life. I needed a girlfriend in my life with whom I could really share myself. There was no one for me to identify and grow with as I began the lessons that would teach me about life, so I could learn about and discover who I really was. Instead, kids would snub, ignore, or tease me. I felt anxiety in all areas: school, relationships and life. It all seemed to be more than I could handle. Evidently it was. That was when my Trichotillomania began.

I remember in seventh grade I was sitting in my fifth period science class. I was anxious about a test I would be taking with my class that day. I never studied much, therefore I wasn't prepared very often, and that added to the chronic anxiety I experienced while in school. I remember feeling like a time bomb ready to explode, and this was to be my explosion.

I hated myself, never feeling like I fit in this world. I began stroking my outer corner eyelashes of my right

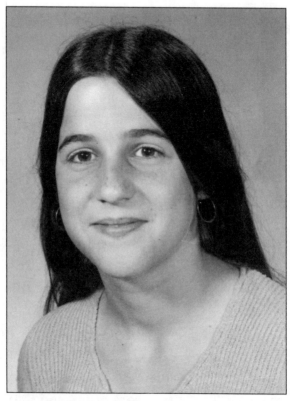

Seventh Grade school picture, a few
months before pulling began.

eye. I pulled lightly, then a little harder, and out came an eyelash. It hurt, but there was also a strange sense of comfort and relief. I ignored the pain and felt again for another eyelash. By the time the test was over, I had pulled out about fifteen eyelashes. Approximately one-eighth of an inch was missing and my eye had swollen noticeably. I was so embarrassed. I now looked physically how I had felt always felt internally. Classmates were not shy about telling me how weird I was for doing that.

My last class of the day was Student Government. I was literally surrounded by all the popular people of the school. I knew I didn't fit in, but I hoped that I might become part of the group. If I were in the class with them, maybe they would come to like me.

This class was already uncomfortable for me, because I was the school secretary only by forfeit. The girl who had won that position had to step down. She was one of the hardest "chicks" in school. Most people were afraid of her, but they still chose her over me to be secretary! This illustrates very clearly just how unpopular I was.

So there I sat, with kids actually hovering over me, asking what happened to my eye. I felt so ashamed. I went home so devastated. I believe I went right to my parents' room where my mom had some tweezers (because I didn't have any at that point). I was all alone, and I kept pulling, very methodically, as if thinning out the lashes would make it look less obvious. (What was I thinking?) Anyhow, I tried to correct my mistake, and plucked out more eyelashes. By this time, I was now drawn into the obsession of pulling.

I remember feeling like I wanted my hands handcuffed. I wanted to break my fingers and break both of my arms. I tried chewing my fingernails down to the cuticle so that they'd be too sore to pull.

One day, not long after that, I got the "brilliant" idea to pull out my thick eyebrows instead, so I would not pull out my eyelashes anymore. Unfortunately, I was very mistaken.

I remember laying on the family room couch alone watching television, as I always did when I came home after school. I pulled the drapes so the room would be completely dark, and made sure the door was shut so that no one would come in and bother me. Then I began plucking out my eyebrows with my fingers.

I started in the inside corner of my thick eyebrows, closest to my nose. It felt good and I felt like I could, that I had plenty to spare. I had no idea that I was creating another problem. I just kept pulling.

Next I began to pull on the outside edges of my eyebrows, doing a symmetric type of thing on both sides. Then I would feel my eyebrows to try to picture

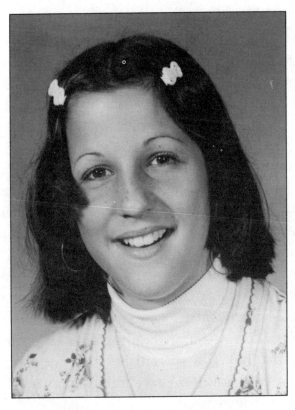

Eighth Grade School Picture

in my head what they looked like. I got up and went into my bathroom When I looked in the mirror, I saw the same shape as Groucho Marx's very rectangular boxy eyebrows. I was devastated. I felt very lost at that point, because I had now ruined another part of myself and I knew that I had dug my "hole" deeper.

I tried to figure out how to solve this problem. I began tweezing my eyebrows one by one. (I wish I had known then, like I do now, how to apply eyebrow pencil to look natural.) I felt it would look more peculiar if I drew in the spaces instead of tweezing them thinner. I felt if I pulled them out and made them look halfway acceptable it would appear that I had meant to, whereas if I drew them in it would be obvious that I had pulled them out. I didn't want to draw any more attention to my "weird" behavior. Penciling in eyebrows was also not the style back then! (Though, nor were thinly plucked eyebrows at my age of twelve, either!) But that's what I did. I ended up tweezing most of my eyebrows out, and I looked awkward because my pencil-thin eyebrows did not fit my face frame or my style. Once again I was devastated.

My self-hate deepened. The feelings of powerlessness terrified me. My life was out of control, and it was very apparent to me that I had a major problem. Unfortunately, no one had ever heard of anyone pulling out their hair before. I felt I was an enigma. I believed I didn't belong anywhere and it was confirmed almost daily because I was the object of much teasing and ridicule.

The rest of my junior high experience is blurry, for I don't have many memories. I believe it was because my life was so painful that I shut down emotionally to survive it.

I do have a few memories that began to emerge these last years of crying in my bed many, many times, due to my pain caused from Trich. I remember my mom trying to comfort me, but unable to help me because she did not know what was the matter with me. I continuously felt very alone and tormented. I couldn't keep my hands away from my face. I was afraid and alone, writhing in self-hatred.

In high school, due to the pressure of not wanting anyone to criticize me for pulling, I would stop pulling out of sheer peer pressure and determination when it was at a noticeable stage.

Halfway into my freshman year I discovered drugs. I liked them because they provided a way for me to not have to feel anymore. They also gave me a sense of euphoria so that I felt okay with myself. (Now I look back and recognize that I, in no way, felt okay with myself. The drugs just made me detach temporarily from my low self-esteem and my anxiety regarding life

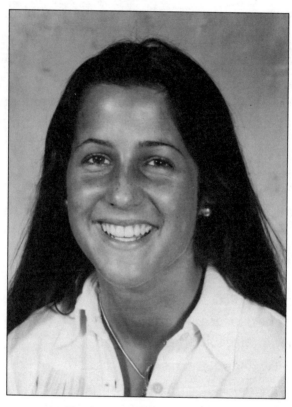

Junior in High School
Lashes and brows!

as a whole.) I was always looking for something to fill the void in myself. Drugs ended up only making it worse.

Once again, the boys' attention made me feel popular and wanted. Unfortunately, as I got older and still possessed no self-esteem, my desire for acceptance cost me physically as well as emotionally. By this time, I didn't hold a strong love or respect for my body, so I inappropriately began to use it to gain popularity.

As I got more into drug use, I eventually lost my virginity. I felt like I had given away my heart and soul. That was the final straw. I didn't care about myself anymore. It was around that time that I first opened myself to God. A group of kids on my campus attended a Christian youth group called "Young Life." They really touched me with their messages from the Bible of God's love, but this only had a limited effect because of my inability to love myself.

In the middle of my junior year of high school I felt, as did my parents, that I needed to get out of the environment I was in. I "graduated" by taking my state's high school proficiency test and went directly into my city's junior college.

I liked college, for the peer pressure seemed to be nonexistent, especially due to its location being in Santa Cruz, California. Most of my classes were of a fun nature. I still felt like I was different from everyone else regarding my pulling, but it felt wonderful not having the peer pressures of high school. I continued to seek spiritual enlightenment through all sorts of avenues, but inside I kept returning to the belief in the God of the Bible.

Due to the lack of peace in my life and my rebellious nature, I still fought my parents on every issue. I was at an age where I was trying to grow up, but really had no idea of how to do it. (But that wasn't going to stop me!)

I ended up getting pregnant, married, and having my first child by the time I was nineteen. Needless to say, due to all the stress in my life and my ability to isolate myself from anyone outside my house, my pulling became the worst it had ever been. Pulling all my eyelashes and eyebrows out wasn't enough. I started pulling my pubic hair, too.

For the most part, I still felt better overall than I ever had in my life. I liked the freedom that came with being an adult. I loved my husband very much (in the capacity that I understood love). He was kind and he loved me regardless of how I looked. Pulling had become my way of releasing tension and I was able to isolate myself in my house when I wanted to feel safe from this world and its people. This seemed to work for me very well, at least for several years.

I felt most uncomfortable about my pulling when I got around other people. I would be very shifty-eyed to avoid eye contact. It was very typical for me to put a distance between myself and other people. What was the hardest for me was when I had to go to my Ob/Gyn doctor visits when I was pregnant. I would go into a major "shame attack" when I'd have to unveil for the doctor during my appointments.

It saddened me most when my due date would be nearing. I would be more nervous about my eye makeup coming off during labor, or making sure no one wiped my eyebrows off, than about the whole labor and delivery process itself.

When the baby was finally born I would actually get up after everyone had left the room to go reapply my makeup. That behavior repeated itself until my third child, Mikaela, was born. It was wonderful to not care how my face endured the labor, or what doctors or nurses thought of my lack of body hair. My focus was on my baby and my joy in her arrival.

Ten years earlier, shortly after the birth of my second daughter, Alyson, I had a strong impression in my mind of a picture, or a vision, of me speaking about my pulling to an auditorium full of people. That was all I saw. I didn't yet know of anyone else who pulled, so I had no impression of whether these people were pullers or not.

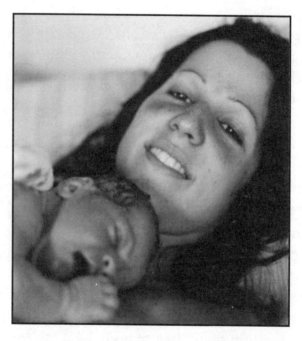

Cheryn after Alyson's birth

I did know for the first time that my life experience with Trich was not going to be in vain. I felt hopeful that something good was going to come from it.

A few years would pass before I'd learn my condition of hair pulling had a name, and that I wasn't alone. It wasn't until I was twenty five years old that I happened to be browsing through an Ann Landers article about a mother whose daughter pulled out her eyelashes. Ann Landers' response was that it was called Trichotillomania, and that a million people do it. (I don't remember the correct quote exactly. The correct answer now in the 1990's is that an estimated six to eight million people have Trichotillomania.) I was stunned.

I still had so much shame in my life around pulling that I just shut the newspaper very quickly. I hoped that no one else would see it because then they would know why I pulled. (I had never talked about it.) I shut the newspaper up, but it was the beginning of my realization that I was not alone. I began to feel a sense of normalcy that I never had felt before. I still felt that I was not part of the norm, but at least there was a name for this "demon" and Ann Landers wrote that it affected millions. (In my mind I immediately discounted millions as not to be taken literally. I felt it had to be a figure of speech, more like a total of one hundred people!)

In the following years I slowly opened up to people, one at a time, and told them my deepest secret. I was terrified of rejection. More than not, the reaction was loving and accepting, but occasionally I'd share with an inappropriate person and I'd get the "weird" look and "ew" response. It would be a few years before I would finally realize that those types of people were the ones with the real problem and that I didn't want people like that in my life.

Thankfully, many people would say that it wasn't a big deal, and that they didn't think of me any differently. That enabled me to begin to look at myself and realize I was okay. I was on the road to recovery and healing.

Some friendships began to develop that offered a safe place for me to learn to be myself. I opened my life up to two women, Rene Strasser and Christina Pearson, who were to become my two dearest women friends. They offered me loving support and no judgment. I learned to get in touch with my feelings and discover who I was. I watched them very closely and saw their honesty with themselves. Slowly I began to explore each aspect of my life with a new respect and honor for myself and my recovery process. I also learned to forgive the mistakes I had made and to try to forgive others. I realized that my unforgiving attitude was only hurting me. I wanted to be free from anger and resentment. (I also recognized that I pulled often because of those negative feelings.)

Rene and Christina were gifts in my life, helping me learn how to love myself unconditionally. Their influence still affects my life today. It soon became easier and easier for me to share with other people. (Unbeknownst to me, it would be through sharing that my shame around hair pulling would someday become nonexistent.)

My self-esteem was beginning to improve. I was feeling acceptance from people I respected and I grew steadily in my recovery, gaining more ability to love, forgive and respect myself.

From 1972 until 1987 I had issues of feeling abandoned by God (regarding my Trichotillomania). I had prayed many prayers for deliverance from this affliction and obsession, and never felt like they had been answered.

I believed that my pulling was a spiritual issue and that I needed deliverance from a demonic power. I was so desperate that I went on a nineteen-day fast of nothing but water in my early twenties after reading a verse in the Bible in Isaiah 58:6. I'm embarrassed to admit that I had even been convinced by some sincere but misguided people to let them try to exorcize me.

I continued to pray many times, over many years experiencing no change. This was one prayer that I believed continued to be unanswered, but inside I felt hope that it wasn't true. I would reaffirm to myself that God was allowing it for some reason, because I knew His presence in my life and had seen many prayers answered. (Years later I would see that God did have a bigger picture and a wonderful plan. He knew the purpose this affliction would play in my life and He had never abandoned me at all.)

My life has felt like a very long and hard road, with many lessons I probably could have avoided if I hadn't been such a strong-willed person who wanted to do things my way. But everything has turned out wonderfully, for which I am very grateful.

I am going to end this chapter with accounts of events I wanted to share with you. My desire is to share my life with you, but it is difficult to try to attempt this within one chapter. So here is a quick overview:

I went through an amicable divorce after ten years of marriage. I am now happily married to my best friend, Michael, who has been a wonderful support in my life. We have added two more children to our family, Mikaela and Michael II.

Rene Strasser introduced me to Christina Pearson, the first person I ever met who had Trichotillomania.

Christina is now the founder and Executive Director of the Trichotillomania Learning Center (see Chapter 12). I am going to go into detail about our meeting because I consider it to be a miracle.

Rene told me she had heard a woman named Christina share about pulling her hair out of her head. I called Christina immediately, and we planned to get together. For several weeks Christina and I tried to get together to talk. We kept missing each other for one reason or another.

She finally called me late one evening and asked me for my address so that she could mail me the information she had received from the Obsessive Compulsive Foundation regarding Trichotillomania. When I told her my address, she gasped. She lived only two houses away from me. (We lived in the Santa Cruz mountains, and that was quite amazing.) We ran out to greet each other in our pajamas and hugged. It was like meeting my long lost twin, for she knew my pain, and I knew hers. At the same time, we both were a little uncomfortable too, but it didn't take long for us to become comfortable. She showed me her bald spots and I removed my makeup completely. (I never had even removed my makeup for my first husband. I slept in my makeup and would awaken early to reapply any missing makeup!)

We talked and cried for a few hours, and spoke of our desires to reach out to the others who were part of our "family" who were still thinking they were the only one. I shared my vision of speaking to others and she shared her desire to start a center, which she went on to do. When it became time for her to go home, I walked her back to her house. As I was walking back to home, some of the neighbors drove by in their car. I waved. Then I passed by a mirror at home, realized to my terror that I had no makeup on, and quickly called Christina. I screamed in terror, "I just passed my neighbor waving and I have no makeup on!" I then began to laugh, because what else could I really do? It was wonderful to have her support, which I never experienced in that way before. I love that story and wanted to share it with you.

In 1991 I got my eyelids tattooed. It was incredibly painful, but well worth it. This allowed me to feel free to cry, rub my eyes, swim, etc. I am not recommending tattooing, though, for this process can be dangerous.

I have attended all four retreats that the Trichotillomania Learning Center has held so far. Around ninety to one-hundred people attend yearly, coming from all parts of the world. Each retreat has brought great healing. I highly recommend attending these retreats.

After the first retreat, I began to write this book. This in itself is quite a miracle, for I couldn't even keep a journal before that. I knew intuitively, however, that there was a book I was supposed to write. I was completely overwhelmed with this, and I quickly turned the book over to God, and said, "You write it through me, if you want it written. I can't!" Then I let it go. I found myself feeling moved with words and ideas and I tried to always write down notes or dictate them into a tape recorder. I would be occasionally unable to sleep at night, as my mind would be full of words that I needed to write. The book took shape, and here it is! I am still amazed! This book truly reflects the actual processing in my recovery. I basically wrote it as I lived it.

After the second retreat, the idea to design a truly natural-looking eyelash came into my mind. From that point on Cheryn International came into existence.

C.I. is a mail-order company which offers a line of products to subtly enhance the beauty of those who have experienced hair loss of various types. My desire was to provide a feeling of beauty and normalcy to people like myself. It now offers a large line of eye makeup and beautiful headwear and guarantees the lowest costs on wigs and hairpieces.

I want to mention events I avoided for fear of discovery, because I know we share many, if not all, of these same experiences.

I avoided crying, eye and dental appointments, swimming and other water activities. (In 1987 I finally got certified as a scuba diver, determined to not allow my Trich to rob me of any more pleasures in my life.)

I did not have a pap smear for eight years, which could have been life-threatening. Chiropractor visits were loathsome, for when I was face down on the table my "eyebrows" would usually be on the paper after the adjustment, instead of on my face. I also didn't like the close encounter when the doctor would adjust my neck.

I had the same problem with hairdressers. When they'd be cutting my hair from the side, I felt very uncomfortable. (What helped was telling them about it first. I felt like I'd rather break the ice myself than imagine them wondering why I had no lashes or eyebrows.)

I began to address my fears, determined to overcome them and their strangulating power. (I did begin small, mind you.) At age twenty five I began by sliding down a "fire pole" at the park. It had always bothered me that I was afraid to do what little kids did all the time. Next I took a self-defense class called "Model Mugging" that was very instrumental in my claiming my worth. I don't know if I can explain why, I just stood up and defended myself in a way I never had, and I grew tremendously in those classes. I next went river rafting and jumped from a rope swing into the river. Both rafting and swinging were huge steps for me. Finally, I was ready for the ultimate test. I went skydiving on my twenty-eighth birthday. The experience was very liberating and empowering. It instilled in me a feeling that I no longer needed to feel oppressed by fear. I no longer want to allow anything to "rip me off" of what life has for me. Life is fun, and I want to live it to its fullest!

Today I love and accept myself. The emotional and physical effects of pulling no longer have the hold on me emotionally or physically that they had in the past. The torment and self-hatred are gone. I still have my relapses of pulling and I imagine that I probably always will, to some degree, but my time of abstinence lengthens between pulling episodes and the duration of time I keep my hair is longer. However, the devastation to my self-esteem and the depression that accompanied my pulling is no longer alive.

The layers of pain have been removed gently, one by one, and I am consistently continuing to grow in awareness. Today I have a lot of patience regarding my recovery. I still get disappointed if I've pulled, but today I realize that I'm working through a process, and it takes time to recover. Every day is a new day, and I am not failing if I slip into my habit. I just have a new opportunity to learn a little bit more about who I am and why I pull.

The changes I have experienced on my journey to recover have been quite different than I had originally thought they would be. I have always thought that my

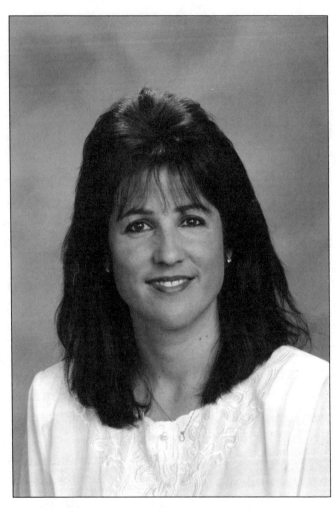

Cheryn Salazar
1995

recovery would be identified only by having my hair back. Now I define recovery as reclaiming myself and restoring my self-esteem, from the inside out, not the reverse. The evidence of my not pulling has stopped being my victory trophy.

If I had the choice to live my life over again, I would choose to live it with Trichotillomania. That is a huge statement and believe me, I am completely aware of what I am saying.

I say this because I have found the hidden treasures in my life that have come from overcoming the devastation caused by Trichotillomania. I embrace all of my trials with faith because they are in my life to teach me. I have not been convinced otherwise. My life reflects my findings. I hope you find the answers to all of your life questions, too.

3

ISOLATION
&
DEPRESSION

When I was reading through hundreds of letters, from people with Trichotillomania or who knew someone with "Trich," I kept seeing a recurring theme of isolation and depression. There was also great sadness, self-disgust and feelings of being weird, to name just a few. Isolation and Trich walked hand in hand in my life. I'm not sure which came first, like the chicken or the egg, but all I know is that once Trich entered my life, I mastered isolation, or rather, it mastered me.

Isolation was not only active in protecting me by pushing away the scary outside world, but it also most devastatingly pushed myself away from me. The natural processes I should have gone through to develop and mature into adulthood were stunted. I was left emotionally handicapped due to the crippling repercussions of isolation.

Isolation was like an ivy that grew wrapping itself around the branches of my emotions, entangling new shoots of growth as if to protect it from a danger, when the danger actually only existed in my mind.

The further I retreated inward, the more withdrawn and afraid I became. I was very needy and always trying to fix myself with different vices like men, food, or drugs.

I never knew of the non-sexual emotional intimacy that two best friends share. Not knowing it even existed, I never sought it. I basically settled for anyone who would like me. I just figured people didn't like me, see worth in me, or want me as their friend. I felt I was empty of value and had nothing to offer. I didn't have any self-esteem. It wasn't until I had a few women friends in my life who were honest with themselves and others (not trying to be perfect) that I began to learn about and experience what friendship is supposed to entail.

I was in my early twenties when I met Jan. She was fun and I sensed an honesty about her, and she liked me just as I was. I liked that. A few years later after I went through some growth changes, I asked her how she felt I used to be. She told me I appeared to her to be loving, but like a robot. (Empty, always seeming to agree with everyone, and never holding my own views.) She was right. I was so afraid of judgment and being different that I would most always agree with everyone. I seldom expressed my own opinions, probably because I really didn't have any confidence. I had felt so different all my life and didn't want to be different ever again. Anyway, as Jan and I got to know each other, I saw her transparency and honesty with herself. I wanted to be like that. It also made me feel safer to begin to look at who I was, whoever and whatever that was! This was the beginning of my long road of self-discovery. I began to break out of the clutches of isolation. I now began to trust someone.

There have been only three adults in my life that have deeply affected me in this way. Rene Strasser, Christina Pearson and my husband Michael Salazar. A few years after knowing Jan, I met my dear friend Rene. She became, and still is, like a sister to me. Rene was the first person I knew who began working to recover, to become healthy emotionally where previously she had not been. Watching her, I got direction and courage to venture out into my own recovery. I recognized my dysfunctional behavior and began reading books and attending support groups for others like myself at Codependents Anonymous. (I'll speak about CoDa later and what it is to be codependent.) I didn't want to live in the parameters I had used before, which were so negative and emotionally harmful. Rene was my sounding board and my validator. She supported me emotionally through many tough times. In fact, through Rene I met Christina Pearson, who was unknowingly my neighbor and future founder of the Trichotillomania Learning Center. Christina was an incredible gift to me. She was the first hair puller I ever met. She became my dear friend and confidante. With Christina I began to emerge from my isolation, feeling nothing but safety and love emanating from her spirit. Never did she judge me. I let her know every deep dark *terrible* secret and she didn't bat an eyelash. (Sorry for the pun!) Christina always let me know I wasn't this terrible person I made myself out to be. I knew I had done some bad things, but knowing I wasn't alone allowed me to emerge. My shame became replaced with love. I recognized that everyone has something with which to contend.

My isolation tomb was broken into. More accurately, once the door was ajar, it slowly began to open up until it was wide open. The process took several years, several good, freeing, nurturing years. Metamorphosis best describes my "caterpillar in a cocoon to butterfly" experience.

My journey has taken me from being a woman who lived in isolation and depression to one living in self-acceptance, forgiveness, and self-love. I am still learning to claim and apply these truths, because for so long I lived to the contrary. Old behaviors can be difficult to change.

I have come to a place of reconciliation with myself. I no longer feel that Trichotillomania is *who* I am, it is just something I *do* when I'm stressed. It is a way for me to release stress, a coping mechanism in my life. One person might chew their nails, another person might use food, another might abuse alcohol, or, of course, any combination of many different dysfunctions. The following are a few more vices used to escape stresses or fill voids: workaholism, compulsive cleaning, drug addiction, sex addiction, compulsive gambling, and shoplifting. Compulsions can manifest themselves in many ways. We all are familiar with these dysfunctions because we have heard about them, but Trichotillomania is still relatively unknown. Thankfully, it is now getting more recognition, but it hasn't until the past few years. There is still more acceptance, if you will, of alcoholism, overeating, etc. People still criticize these conditions and the people who suffer from them, but the conditions are not a peculiarity. It is just an obvious loss of control. Pulling out one's own hair is still considered a peculiarity. Trichotillomania still is met with an "ew," "weird" reaction.

My venture began seven years ago when I read my first self-help book, *Women Who Love Too Much*, by Robin Norwood. I learned a little bit about myself in that book and I began to look at myself in a different light.

I was amazed at how I identified with the women in the book and their scenarios. I began to understand my "love addiction" behavior and my reasons for the inappropriate choices of men I had chosen in my life. I loved to feel love from men, for I felt no love for myself. I needed their love to survive and feel important. Because I couldn't find it in myself, I found it in others, as I did when I was growing up. Of course, this was never a true love. Now I realize that I was in love with feeling loved. I look back now and can see ever so clearly that it never was the person that I loved. They were always as emotionally unhealthy as I was, and incapable of having a healthy relationship. That's why I drew to them!

A sense of relief came over me as I discovered that I wasn't a bad person. I was just a needy and insecure person who wanted to feel loved. I had been choosing men that I felt I could change or help. This made me feel I had significance if I could succeed. It was also because I felt safer to be with a person who was so down and out that they would not leave me. I always chose men who weren't threatening to my self-esteem.

I began questioning my behaviors and choices in life, instead of criticizing myself for them. I started looking at my life experiences in a different perspective, thus discovering another side of myself. This "self-help" opened up a new awareness for me. I began to look inside myself to better understand why I was who I was.

I am still amazed at how much relief came to my inner spirit when I began to let this secret out of the hidden recesses of my being. I began to search for answers to the reasons why I pulled and soon discovered how my self-esteem and emotional makeup had been so damaged by the effects of Trichotillomania.

I have learned a gentleness, a compassion and a love that were foreign to me previously.

At that time I also had a lot of loving support in my life. I developed a network of friends that loved me unconditionally. This provided me with the courage to begin to look for and find the person they saw in me and loved. It always amazed me that anyone could love me.

Each step is worthwhile and beneficial. Just as a steep mountain is tiresome to climb, the elation and reward come throughout the walk, not just at reaching the top.

A few of the many gifts I have received as I have pressed on toward the goal have been that my bouts with depression are decreasing and my perfectionism is being fought and destroyed. I also can say today that I love myself. I never ever could say that before I began this journey.

My hope for you is that I have encouraged you to reach out of your isolation and unlock the door and let it swing open. I believe once we step onto the path of recovery, the pathway itself will guide our next step and the rest of the following steps to self-discovery. It takes truthful, positive affirmations to replace the negative ones perhaps fed to us by those who have had influence in our life. We need to retrain our mind, refusing and replacing the false negative messages.

Instead, learn to recognize and realize your true value. You are precious and wonderfully made. You are valuable.

I used to commit a continual silent suicide inside myself. Today I love life and can say "I love myself." Please, if you see yourself in my story, begin to learn to understand yourself. Identify the developmental stages in your childhood and upbringing that might have contributed to or caused the dysfunctions in your life today. If they remain unrevealed and unaddressed, they will remain. You will continue to be the same.

You have the opportunity, if you choose, to "represent" your inner child that was, for whatever reason, not given the tools to live in this world and to "reparent" her/him. You can, as many already have, change and come to love yourself and see yourself as precious and valuable.

You might need to change your environment, whom you are around, and stop using mind altering substances which keep you shut down and emotionally isolated. Sobriety and AA soon accompanied me in my quest for emotional recovery. Big leaps were made when I quit drinking. Looking back, I see how necessary sobriety was in enabling me to make changes and continue growing.

Also, if your mate or loved ones harass you, I would encourage you to set boundaries. Don't accept inappropriate behavior from them. As you set these boundaries, I believe your self-respect and sense of value will increase, and you will no longer be able or willing to tolerate this negative behavior.

I have struggled with depression as long as I can remember. I believe that my insecurities and absence of self-love contributed to many bouts. Here is a journal entry of one of my depressions. It was written with other pullers in my thoughts.

Journal entry from 1994

Isolation and depression, most of the time, go hand in hand for me. Lately I have been experiencing depression to a degree I haven't felt in a long time. Last night my husband told me that during and after a pulling episode I push him away. I began to cry because I realized that I push everyone away. The place I go to is such a lonely place. Then I felt frustration for having to experience this depth of pain. I am so tired of the loneliness that comes from feeling my pain at this depth that my husband can't share. I feel like there would be some comfort if he could touch the parts of me that are in agony, if he could relate to the disappointment I feel after pulling. I'm sure he's had his own troubles in his life, but these are mine (yours and mine). You still can't really help me except by understanding, and maybe crying with me. I am so grateful that you understand my pain, but right now it still doesn't seem like that is enough. I feel like a car accident victim who has lost my face in an accident, and in the hospital there are other disfigured patients who understand, but I'm still on my own to feel my pain. My true comfort is that I know that God understands me and is there for me. When I surrender myself and my pain to Him, I feel touched. Hope and peace replace my pain.

But I have isolated myself since I was twelve, so sometimes I forget to reach out of myself and get comfort. Sometimes Mike can connect with me in such a way that helps, if I am able to really let go and cry from my inner depths. Right now I am just angry at Trichotillomania for its devastating repercussions. I notice that my children also suffer from my isolation. One sign is that they become needy or restless. When I am isolating myself, I am less patient and I want to be alone. I believe that the role of the mother is that of a hubcap on a wheel; we keep the emotional well-being of the family together. It bothers me very much that my pulling hurts my husband and my children. I am tired of the battle and really desire to reach the point of full love for myself where I don't push myself or other people away anymore.

One night I saw a woman singing at a coffee house. She was beautiful in a nonphysical way. She has the gift of being a storyteller and her songs are powerful, deep and moving. What drew me to this woman was the inner beauty she possessed. When she was eight, she had the traumatic experience of being bitten in the face by a dog. She had been a new student in her school, having just moved there shortly before her accident. She had no friends. She had just left a wonderful neighborhood of her best friends and her childhood home. She says that experience shaped her life. Her new nickname was "Scarface." She believed the children's taunts. She suffered in a way I understood. But her beauty and her faith were all I saw when I looked at her. She shined. She had overcome. She loved. I knew that more than lashes and eyebrows I wanted peace with how I looked, who I was without these hairs on my face. I wanted that depth of acceptance, which she said came for her after much soul-searching and hard work. I knew I'd have to fight for my "self."

The search was on. In a society that measures one's value by their outer appearance, I had to find a deeper, different reality. I had gone through a certain amount of growth already that brought me to a certain depth and realization, so I knew this was the true pathway and reality that I wanted. But in that coffeehouse when Sally was singing, I realized I still had a closed fist around certain areas of my self-esteem in my heart which had not yet been penetrated and healed. I really saw the devastation of this when Mike was telling me how he saw my personality change when I've been pulling, and that isolation and depression always follow. I think I saw it clearer than ever that night. There were some deep changes that needed to be addressed. I saw that Trich was still damaging me and traumatizing my life. I'd had enough. This had to stop. I wasn't willing to be robbed anymore.

What I find very ironic is that something so devastating would bring forth a new, better life for me. As much as I hated Trich, it had become my ally in the process. This is like a hurricane that comes through an old, tattered town and devastates everything there. The government emergency aid comes and gives the poor town a face-lift which ends up making it functional in a way it had never been. Tourists begin to stop there, to see the pictures of how it was before, and they see the shops, homes and landscapes of today. The quality of life has improved for the townspeople, but not without a lot of work.

When I change my outlook beginning on the inside, I always seem to get a clearer perspective. (Sometimes

I'll write a list of things that I am grateful for.) I believe that we can all do this. We *must* do this in order to live a quality life that isn't immersed in self-pity.

One of my favorite examples of someone living a quality life is of a quadriplegic woman named Joni Eareckson Tada who touched my life around fifteen years ago. I read one of her books and was amazed at her life story.

She had been an active teenager, popular and pretty, who broke her neck and became paralyzed after diving into the shallow area of a swimming hole. Never believing that she'd have quality of life again, she wished for death. As she went through much physical and emotional tragedy, she came to surrender her life and heart to her circumstances. Because of everything she was able to learn from her difficult experiences due to her injury and paralysis, Joni said that if she had a choice to live life over again, she would choose to live this one just as it has been. Her story is quite uplifting, amazing and inspirational. Who would have thought that anyone could ever find good in such a terrible situation? She has become an accomplished artist who paints and draws, using her teeth to hold her brushes and pencils. Joni has also recorded several Christian music albums, and has been married to a wonderful man named Ken Tada for over a decade.

64

Her surrender to God and His faithfulness in her life is inspiring. Her book tells of her pain, suffering, and anger, and reading them would probably make anyone else thankful for their situation. It's included in my "Suggested Reading" segment in the back of this book.

If I were to have a choice to live my life over again, I, too, feel that I would definitely choose to go through my life again with Trich. As much as I hate pain and discomfort, I have found that if it weren't for the lessons I have learned through Trichotillomania, I would not have gotten to the place I am in my life today. I have received many blessings also in helping others with Trichotillomania. I have found a richness in discovering myself in ways I never knew existed. Life is truly rich and beautiful, and I believe every circumstance happens for a reason. My faith gives me tremendous peace, for I know that every circumstance given to me in my life has not been random. Instead it is an opportunity for me to grow. I certainly have grown from Trichotillomania and become better from it. Today I completely accept it and truly am grateful for what it has taught me. That doesn't mean I love not having lashes and eyebrows. It means I value more than hair the many things I have learned from it.

❧ 4 ❧

IDENTIFYING
& DIFFUSING
SHAME, ANXIETIES
& EMOTIONS

In the previous chapter I mentioned shame reduction as a key point to recovering. This issue is so prevalent and powerful that I chose to write a chapter on it, along with addressing anxieties and emotions.

Sharing diffuses shame. The most comfortable and safest environments that I have been in when I have shared were in a Trich support group or talking with my best friend. Where and who you choose to talk to need to be decided by you alone, but I encourage you to talk with someone you can trust, with whom you can open up this secretive area of your life. The more light that is brought into these dark places, the more release from shame will occur because then the fears and anxieties will begin to relinquish. This is an example of the process I mentioned in the introduction of this book: putting the key in the door and letting the process unfold for us.

YOU ARE DEFINITELY NOT ALONE

The most recent statistics tell us that 2 percent of our population, six to eight million people in the United States alone, experience Trichotillomania.

That is probably as surprising to you as it was to me. Only in recent years has the medical field been made aware of Trichotillomania and its many sufferers. There were no calculations and no studies due to a lack of awareness of our condition, for most "Trichsters" are quite proficient at hiding their condition. Only since many sufferers began "coming out of the closet" has the magnitude of this disorder been discovered, by both the medical profession as well as ourselves.

We know that hair pulling has been in existence for a long time. In the Old Testament there was a prophet named Ezra who pulled out his hair and beard. In Ezra 9:3, Ezra said, " . . . and when I heard this thing, I rent my garment and my mantle, and plucked off the hair of my head and of my beard." Also, Trichotillomania rumors include that Cleopatra also pulled her hair out and wore a wig. The point is, you and I are far from being alone in this disorder, and it certainly is not new.

The statement, "You are not alone" has become my comfort as well as my book's title. There is such a strong desire in my heart to get this message out to everyone who suffers with Trich. The feeling of being the only one (and the stigma of being weird or crazy that seems to accompany each one of us) is devastating. I believe that feeling has been equally as damaging and debilitating as the actual act of pulling and its aftereffects. I know that when I discovered I wasn't alone, the healing process began in me. My hope is that it helps you, too.

One area which needed healing was the harmful impression that I was different. I have noticed that in my years of growing up, I have gone to some extreme measures to not feel different, look different, or be different from anyone else. Until around age twenty-seven I really had no concept of who I was, because I felt so odd and unlovable. I still don't quite understand why I felt so unfavorably toward myself. I seemed to buy into many of my peers' taunts and made them my own. Anyhow, as I was growing up into adulthood, I seldom gave an opposing view because I was very unsure of what my perspectives were. I didn't want anyone else to think that I was different, for that was my greatest fear.

Anytime other people looked at me, I felt uncomfortable. For example, being the right weight or having long eyelashes seemed to draw more looks from guys than if I were chubby or lashless. I'd always seem to sabotage myself and then wonder why I couldn't allow myself to feel attractive. I felt uncomfortable if I were at my right weight because then I'd receive more attention, so I'd subconsciously regain the weight I had just worked to lose. Very often when I would have most all of my eyelashes in, I would then pull them out. I never understood why, then, but now I believe that I didn't want to be more attractive than another person and I wanted to blend in. I didn't want to be different.

I still have trouble receiving a compliment easily. If someone says I'm looking good, I most often quip back with a "well, you haven't seen me naked" type of joking. I have a hard time with compliments on my outer appearance. I recognize that there is no worth in it. I also seem to either be at my right weight and lashless or browless, or I am overweight and have lashes or brows. I used to think it was because I felt uncomfortable if things were going too well for me, which maybe was true before. (There was a lot of inner turmoil and drama in my life as a child growing up, and drama was normal for me. So I'd just create drama when things were good.) Today I believe it is because I need to have some sort of outlet when I'm stressed or anxious.

As I heard of other people's nervous problems, I was able to see enough similarity to my own that I realized I was ordinary, or at least not as unusual as I thought! I had an errant sense of shame about myself. I had created a picture, a false sense of reality as I was growing up, that other people had it all together. I now know that this was inaccurate. My friendships never possessed the honesty and trust necessary to share each other's personal life experiences.

I heartily believe in sharing and being honest in my friendships. I believe it isn't a true relationship unless you are transparent with each other. After much work, my marriage is like this. It didn't begin this way. At one point we made a decision to have complete honesty toward each other, about ourselves and our feelings. It was a breakthrough for each of us. Sharing is powerful because it diffuses shame. Of course, I would not suggest that you share with an unsafe or inappropriate person. My definition of unsafe is someone who would judge you or criticize you, and doesn't possess an honesty with themselves and their own life. No one has that right, since we all make mistakes. Our life is our life, and our past is our past.

My anxiety level has always been high. Having an "on edge" chemistry and questioning my mental well-being left me always wondering if I were normal. I knew of no one else who pulled out their hair, so that was "strike one" towards me feeling different.

I felt everyone else seemed to have it all together and I knew that was far from true for me. I had a very difficult time doing simple, basic things. Basic chores of a wife and mother were very overwhelming to me. No one else I knew seemed to experience this. "Strike two." It would be many years before I would come to know people who would be honest with me, revealing their own inadequacies and fears. Once I began to discover how I was not alone, I began to be released and healed from the shame that gripped me.

I have heard of many pullers whose parents responded to their child's pulling by one or more of the following behaviors: shaming, hitting, punishing, disgust, and shaving heads (girls as well as boys). If you have experienced any of these behaviors, be aware that you were wronged. I believe you first need to forgive in order to heal, but I might be wrong, for I have never experienced this type of behavior from my parents. I do believe that you need to realize that you were shamed then you need to recover by reparenting your inner child from the past. Forgiving those who have brought you harm will release you from the damaging consequences of anger, hatred and resentment.

No person belongs in your life if they are going to be a voice of shame. Once I set that boundary, I then began to work very hard to remove that voice in my own head. Emotions, if not healthy, can mislead us into doing things we think can help us feel better, but actually are harmful, like pulling hair to relieve an anxiety. You think it is that particular hair that's bothering you, when actually it is some buried emotion from the day or from the past that is causing anxiety. When we don't identify the emotion, we are left with a need to attach the anxiety onto something else. In our case, it is very often our body hair.

Until we learn how to identify our source of anxiety, we will stuff down the problem and focus on a pseudo problem. We never step out of the painful patterns that keep us stuck in so many ways, not just in pulling.

The following article on "Toxic Shame" explains appropriate and inappropriate shame. Understanding and applying this information will help you to heal from the effects you may have experienced in your life from unhealthy shame. (I have marked my additional comments with an asterisk.)

TOXIC SHAME:
Its Origins, Uses, Shame-Binds,
and How to Heal It
by Carl Paul Alasko, PhD, MFCC.

Traditional psychology talks very little about shame. It wasn't until the 1980's, with the work of John Bradshaw and Pia Mellody, among others, that shame started being described as a major therapeutic and social issue. This paper outlines and describes general themes about shame. For more detailed information, read John Bradshaw's book, *Healing the Shame That Binds You*, and Pia Mellody's book, *Facing Co-dependence*.

There are two types of shame: healthy and toxic.

Healthy shame is essential for modesty and good manners. Very little goes a long way. Healthy shame keeps us from offending others. It is very similar to **embarrassment**, though sometimes stronger.

The best way to identify toxic shame is how it feels: bad, useless, empty, worthless, defective, no-good, incapable, less-valuable-than-others, etc. (Unless otherwise specified, the word shame refers to toxic shame.)

—TOXIC shame feels like you ARE a mistake, that you as a person are defective, useless, wrong.

—HEALTHY shame feels like you MADE a mistake. It helps you recognize BEHAVIOR that's incorrect. (Shame is connected to guilt, which you feel when you did or did not DO something.) If you frequently feel guilt that you can't work through, you're probably feeling toxic shame.

(* *I believe shame is what you feel when you are something wrong, and guilt is what you feel when you have done something wrong.*)

Shame must initially come from other people.

Children cannot—while still young—shame themselves. They are, by design, accepting of their mistakes. It's ALWAYS parents, relatives and especially teachers that shame children, using statements that teach children to view themselves as no-good, useless, defective, incapable, etc.

Some common shaming statements (Note that sarcasm is also very shaming): "You'll never learn." "How many times have I already told you?" "What's the matter, you blind?" "If I let you do it, it'll never get done." "Oh, great job!!" (said sarcastically), etc.

The category for boys: "You sissy!" "Cry baby . . . Wimp. . . " "Only girls act that way . . . "

For girls (often subtler, shaming her gender): "We'll ask a boy to help." "You are just a girl." "You have to look pretty." "Young ladies don't do . . . "

Because children are designed to learn, they absorb shaming messages quickly. Depending on the authority of the person using them, the child accepts them as true. Then the shaming message becomes part of the child's "internal" structure or belief system. Subsequently, the child repeats to him/herself the same messages. This is the beginning of low self-esteem. And

a life-long struggle with self-image and self-sabotage.

Shame in society: It's society's most powerful tool. It controls people and classes. It allows more aggressive, stronger people to convince less endowed ones that they DESERVE to be exploited. "I have more because you don't deserve it. You are less valuable than me." It allows one race or ethnic group to exploit (or kill) another. Shame **de-humanizes.**

Shame in the family: Shame very effectively controls others, especially children. Even today it's the most common method of child "discipline." Beating/spanking* children is shaming because it treats their body and feelings as unimportant. (*Author adds, "inappropriately or abusively used.")* Violence tells a child that, "You're not capable of understanding words so I'll use violence and terror to control you." Any violence between a stronger and weaker person is intensely shaming.

Shame in relationships: Shaming other persons "puts them down," lower than yourself, and *more* *subject to control.* Therefore, without doing any self-discipline or "work" on yourself, you can feel better than the other. This is a major dynamic in all interpersonal relationships.

Shame-Binds: Shame is a unique emotion because it "attaches" or binds to all other feelings and behaviors. Examples: Johnny, age six, gets hurt and cries. Dad calls him a cry-baby, or otherwise makes fun of him. Johnny feels shame (worthless in his father's eyes) for feeling and doing something "boys don't do." In the future he'll avoid "female" feelings, perhaps becoming tough and hyper-macho to avoid any feelings of shame. Johnny has a "shame-feeling" bind.

Becky's mom is depressed and/or sick. She says Becky's selfish for asking for something she needs. "All you do is think of yourself!" Thereafter Becky feels shame whenever she tries to ask for something or take care of her needs. To avoid feeling worthless, no-good, selfish, etc., she becomes "needless," taking care of others' needs instead. Becky has a "shame-needs" bind.

A shame-bind maintains dysfunctional beliefs and feelings by activating the feelings of being bad, useless, etc. whenever the shamed activity or feeling is re-experienced. As an adult, John says he doesn't have feelings of pain or fear. In reality, he feels shame whenever he thinks of feeling something not rigidly masculine. Becky feels worthless, bad, useless, whenever she tries to take care of her own needs. She's being selfish! Or she's not assertive in her career because she believes she shouldn't push herself forward. And she feels "bad" when she does so.

There are numerous potential shame-binds: shame-anger, shame-fear, shame-ignorance, shame-existence. . . etc. This is why shame is such a debilitating toxic feeling.

How to heal shame: (These steps are only an outline and are not intended as a substitute for competent professional therapy. If you experience difficulty, please get professional help.)

1. Become aware of how shame feels in your body. Write notes about when you feel useless, empty, defective, etc. How often and how strong are these feelings?

2. Make notes about which circumstances trigger a "shame attack," which is the experience of being overwhelmed by feeling worthless, etc. A shame attack can be so powerful that you become numb,

or you may want to isolate and go to sleep. Or you may experience shame as a generalized feeling of inadequacy that stifles your initiative and joy.

3. Review your family-of-origin history to determine when and how your parents, relatives, teachers shamed you. What did they say and do? Remember: NEGLECT is a powerful source of shame because the message is you're not worth taking care of! Shaming does not have to be overt. It can also be learned by example, i.e., a depressed parent. Writing helps!

4. It is very *helpful* to discuss these events with a close trusted friend or therapist.

5. Then write out a series of affirmative statements that counteract the feelings of shame. Examples: John, (in the above example) would write out: "I have a right to experience all of my feelings." Becky could write: "I have a right to take care of my needs," and so forth.

It's essential to continually confront the feelings of worthlessness, inadequacy, etc. as they appear. Recognize that *you do not deserve* these feelings, they've been "dumped" on you by others. Continued attention to this process is one of the best ways to relieve yourself of toxic shame.

Then you must develop your "boundaries" so that others cannot invade your emotional space at will, and continue to shame you. In some cases you may have to discontinue a relationship based on shame. Certain activities (alcohol, drugs, sex, gambling, violence, etc.) continue the shame cycle. By doing your own difficult and self-disciplined growth work, you can exit from the shame-cycle.

It is also essential to make a commitment to not shame other people, especially children.

(Reprinted by permission.)

How do you address an issue when the issue seems to be surrounded by a circle of impenetrable fog? When I feel like pulling, or am in the midst of it, I am usually unaware of the exact reason why. If there is an overwhelming anxiety behind it, if I feel unable to identify and address what the "eye of the tornado" is, my pulling provides an escape. It's a place of refuge when I am anxious, which I best describe as "zoning out."

I would much rather be able to address what is causing the emotional upset and not pull; however, if I feel unable to do this, I try to begin by addressing one issue at a time, trying to reach the core problem. I picture the process like the peeling of an onion, one layer at a time, because tears are often shed with each layer removed.

I believe many of us share similar behaviors with the bulimic (one who feels the need to purge themselves of their food). They vomit around their feelings, where we instead pull around ours. Let me explain.

I have heard bulimia described as the need to purge because they have ingested someone else's opinions of who they are! They intermesh people's issues and opinions and digest them, later needing to purge by throwing them up, using laxatives or dieting, purging the event or situation from their bodies.

I view Trichotillomania as trying to peel away a concept, situation or experience from one's body. Sexual abuse, criticism, and verbal abuse can peel away at one's own person, altering and transforming them. However, as bulimics soon discover, an unhealthy attempt to escape this abuse can become obsessive, abusive and addictive, leaving one feeling different and freakish. Isn't that the same with us?

Much as I have used the picture of peeling the onion layer by layer in recovery, I personally believe this is often the Trich sufferer's purpose, (intuitively), for lack of knowing another way. The "peeling" off of each eyelash one at a time relieves my anxiety for the moment, but later multiplies my anxiety tenfold.

There were many times I pulled when I was going through an attack of shame, where I had "ingested" someone else's opinions of who I was!

When I began to search for why I pulled my hairs, I began to realize that there were many reasons. To identify them seemed impossible. Perhaps, I felt, if I could just identify my anxieties, or what was going on emotionally when I pulled, then I might be able to unfold this mystery. I do believe that this is the first step that must be taken before the hair puller can recover. The common thread we share, I believe, is that of high anxiety and stress, and a feeling of confusion about why and when we pull.

I have been able to narrow down some of the emotions which influence my inclination to pull. Some are:

- Anxieties of the past, brought up on "old tape" by some happenstance in the day.

- Anxieties of the future. Trying to control, when in fact I am powerless.

- When my chemistry is thrown off, for any number of reasons, for example: PMS, sugar, caffeine (i.e., chocolate, coffee and tea).

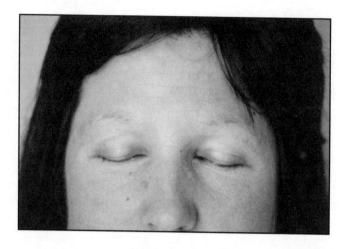

Before Makeup
(I have a slight amount of faded tattooing
on my eyelids. It fades over the years.)

Question: Can we change our chemistry when we are being controlled by our body's natural anxieties? Can we exercise and omit the caffeine and sugar, and find relief? I believe the answer is, "Yes!" Can we listen to relaxation tapes or use relaxation techniques to relieve our compulsions and change the neurological chemistry in our brain? Can we address the issues when they are identifiable and thus alleviate anxiety? For example, if someone hurts our feelings and is abusive or unfair, can we relieve our self-destructive inclinations by getting in touch with how we feel and expressing it, thus taking care of ourselves? I believe so.

As I learn to love myself unconditionally, my pulling decreases. When I take care of myself and don't allow someone to abuse me emotionally, or take advantage of me, or be inappropriate in any way to me, then the urge to pull is lessened or diminished. If I cry when I am sad, mad, hurt, or full of an anxiety that I can't identify, then I feel the tension leave my body. I am more able to feel and address the real issue, and I most often don't feel the need to pull anymore, or I am more able to resist.

Unfortunately, I believe one of the things that a hair puller has a difficult time doing is crying. For me it definitely was, because I couldn't touch on that emotion easily. I had stuffed down my feelings for so long. When I realized that there were many issues in my life that I had never dealt with, I became willing to take whatever steps were necessary to not stuff my feelings anymore.

This meant for me to stop drinking first, for I had used alcohol to release my anxiety. It was an artificial substitute that would only produce an artificial result. The day after drinking I usually felt like I had experienced unwinding or release of built-up stress. But I was truly only covering up the problem, and each time these inner feelings would try to erupt I would go out drinking again. The vicious cycle would continue. I never felt uncomfortable enough to really cry, but I would feel uncomfortable enough to keep pulling.

When I stopped drinking, I became sober in more ways than one. I remember the day I stopped, it was as if the world took on a new look. I felt I was looking at my life with eyes that wanted to see reality. I didn't want to be blinded to it anymore. Drinking and pulling were keeping me from functioning, and I was desperate to become a functioning person. I can really see today how my pulling had affected my daily life, my emotional makeup, my self-esteem, and much more. Quitting drinking was no sweat compared to quitting pulling.

How much do the issues of anxiety affect your pulling? If you could avoid the web of anxiety, could you delete the impulse to pull? I am definitely finding that the answer for me, more and more, is "Yes!"

My emotions have become more level and stable as the anxiety is lessened and my shame is gone about 95 percent. Ever so often, out of the blue, I will experience a day where I'll feel a cloud of shame. I find myself feeling lesser than other people, intimidated, or uncomfortable in my own skin. When this happens, I recognize it and confront it as a lie. Once I have recognized its presence, I then am able to push it away with the truths of affirmation and love, reminding myself of my value.

Our society has always followed trends and styles, being swept one way and the other like the wind. We need to recognize that we don't need to follow trends and styles. We need to learn how we want to dress and look. If we are handicapped it doesn't make us any less of a person, and I think that is very, very important to comprehend in order to be able to realize how whole you are, how you are enough.

I believe that we no longer need to feel isolated as if we are different from our society's norm. We need to realize that everyone has something to contend with, no matter how good they look on the outside. In fact, I believe the more attractive someone looks, the easier they can hide, putting their self-esteem in superficial qualities based on our society's value system.

If I hadn't learned where true beauty lies, I never would have found out who I truly am inside. I know that this search for my inner beauty was prompted by my Trichotillomania. I know in my past, before I began pulling, I was very attractive without any makeup and I based my identity mostly on my appearance. With Trichotillomania, I could put the makeup on and look good, but I knew how I looked without it. So, therefore, what I look like on the outside holds much less importance for me and I am grateful for this. I recognize very clearly that society is disillusioned with the importance of someone's outside appearance and image, and I no longer am influenced by it.

I believe our society and the media have played a big part in influencing one's worth by superficial measurements, thus creating low self-esteem if you do not look like the "perfect picture." We know what that feels like, don't we! However, I feel it is time to recognize our equality, worth and significance.

I see a wonderful strength in people who experience Trichotillomania. We pull, we hope, we pull again, we keep hoping time and time again, and we work hard to overcome our discouragement with each occurrence. There is a saying, "What doesn't kill you strengthens you." I can relate. We are strong people. We must learn to love, accept, and take care of ourselves.

5

CODEPENDENCY
&
POSITIVE
AFFIRMATIONS

This chapter will explain codependency and help you recognize whether it is a part of your life, and if so, how to recover from it. I first heard of codependency in an Alcoholics Anonymous meeting.

This chapter is also a compilation of people's writings, some credited, some anonymous or unknown, which give messages that have helped me and I believe will help you in recognizing and claiming the valuable person that you are. I have gathered them from meetings I have attended since 1989. They have helped me in my recovery from codependency and low self-esteem. Now I am excited to be able to offer them to you, to help equip you, too. I hope that you will be able to apply them to your life to help you on your road of recovery. Remember that recovery is not a destination, but a way of transportation. Let me first begin by giving a definition of codependency.

WHAT IS CODEPENDENCY?

Codependency is difficult to explain in a few sentences. Pia Mellody in her book *Facing Codependency* explains codependency and offers solutions that have helped me and many others reclaim their lives.

My dear friend, Rene Strasser, told me a definition that someone had once given her. She said, "When your life flashes before you and it's someone else's, chances are you're codependent." In other words, when you live your life for someone else, and your identity is in someone else, you are codependent. The definition is really much more involved, and I encourage you to read Pia's book to gain better understanding.

The following patterns and characteristics are offered as a tool to aid in self-evaluation. They may be particularly helpful to newcomers as they begin to understand codependence and may aid those who have been in recovery a while in determining what traits still need attention and transformation. I picked them up at a CoDa meeting in 1989. The portions marked with an asterisk are my additions.

DENIAL PATTERNS:

◆ I have difficulty identifying what I am feeling.

◆ I minimize, alter or deny how I truly feel.

◆ I perceive myself as completely unselfish and dedicated to the well-being of others.
  (* *I am extremely negative toward life/people/ circumstances.*)

LOW SELF-ESTEEM PATTERNS:

◆ I have difficulty making decisions.

◆ I judge everything I think, say or do harshly, as never "good enough."

◆ I am embarrassed to receive recognition and praise or gifts.

◆ I do not ask others to meet my needs or desires.
(* *I am embarrassed by who I am.*)
(* *If they really knew who I was, they wouldn't like me.*)

◆ I value others' approval of my thinking, feelings and behaviors over my own.

◆ I do not perceive myself as a lovable or worthwhile person.

COMPLIANCE PATTERNS:

(* All about how our fears are manifest.)

♦ I compromise my own values and integrity to avoid rejection or others' anger.

♦ I am very sensitive to how others are feeling and feel the same.

(* I feel responsible for others' feelings, such as sadness, happiness, or anger.)

♦ I am extremely loyal, remaining in harmful situations too long.

(* I rescue because I need to be rescued!)

♦ I value others' opinions and feelings more than my own and am often afraid to express differing opinions and feelings of my own.

(* I fear rejection and believe I can't live without their approval and love.)

♦ I put aside my own interests and hobbies in order to do what others want.

(* I can't afford to lose them and take a chance at independence.)

◆ I accept sex when I want love.

(* I reject and neglect my own needs—replacing sex with intimacy.)

CONTROL PATTERNS:
(* These stem from our compliance patterns.)

◆ I believe most other people are incapable of taking care of themselves.
(* I will show them how it's done "right.")

◆ I attempt to convince others of what they "should" think and how they "truly" feel.
(* Fearful of exposing my own needs, I don't allow them to have needs.)

◆ I become resentful when others will not let me help them.
(* I don't know who I am if I'm not needed.)

◆ I freely offer others advice and directions without being asked.
(* I am overly opinionated, or overly passive.)

◆ I lavish gifts and favors on those I care about.
(* Then I get angry when they don't do what I want.)

◆ I use sex to gain approval and acceptance.

◆ I have to be "needed" in order to have a relationship with others.

(Author unknown, reprinted with permission of AlAnon.)

The following, "Signs of Unhealthy Boundaries," is more literature I collected at a CoDa meeting. I possessed most of these signs, but reading them helped me to recognize them in my life. I then began to work on addressing, with the goal of eliminating, each sign one by one. Remember to always be gentle with yourself in your process of recovery.

SIGNS OF UNHEALTHY BOUNDARIES

- Telling all.

- Talk at an intimate level at the first meeting.

- Falling in love with a new acquaintance.

- Falling in love with anyone who reaches out.

- Being overwhelmed by a person—preoccupied.

- Acting on the first sexual impulse.

- Being sexual for your partner, not yourself.

- Going against personal values of rights to please others.

- Not noticing when someone else displays inappropriate boundaries.

- Not noticing when someone invades your boundaries.

- Accepting food, gifts, touch, or sex that you don't want.

- Touching a person without asking.

- Taking as much as you can get for the sake of getting.

- Giving as much as you can give for the sake of giving.

- Allowing someone to take as much as they can from you.

- Letting others direct your life.

- Letting others describe your reality.

- Letting others define you.

- Believing others can anticipate your needs.

- Expecting others to fill your needs automatically.

- Falling apart so someone will take care of you.

- Self-abuse.

- Sexual and physical abuse.

- Food and chemical abuse.

    (Author unknown, reprinted by permission of AlAnon.)

POSITIVE AFFIRMATIONS

What goes in must come out. I believe this is a natural law of life ignored in many situations in our society. A few I think of are our diet, television and movie viewing, alcohol and drug intake, and the choice of company we keep. How can we imagine that we can think negatively and do negative things with no resulting repercussions? We need to replace the negative messages we have received in our life with positive messages, or affirmations. I believe this is how we can change ourselves inwardly and live in an element of peace. I like to describe these positive messages as "the truth," thus believing the negative, harmful messages to be "lies." Out of the abundance of the heart the mouth speaks. Watch your messages and learn from them.

Positive affirmations are absolutely necessary in learning how to diffuse anxiety. The practice of using positive input to replace the negative ingrained messages of our youth and adulthood is quite powerful and effective.

What is a positive affirmation? A positive affirmation is a statement of a loving, positive nature you tell yourself in times of low self-esteem to replace the negative messages you have received in your life.

Another kind of positive affirmation is physical affirmation. When I exercise, I am giving my body a positive message. I not only have endorphins that speak to my body, but I feel better about my body after exercise, even if it is simply a walk around the block. Fresh air and sunshine are very positive for the body. It is very important to find activities and environments that will nurture you, so you can provide yourself with a lifestyle that promotes positive physical affirmations.

My success over pulling comes and goes, depending on how I handle myself when I am feeling stress. If I am not able to diffuse my physical anxiety (usually by crying or exercising), then I usually cannot resist the temptation to pull. Pulling is the most convenient catalyst for me to relax, so it takes my effort to choose a more productive way. However, I don't always have the mind-set to motivate myself to get past my circumstances and do what I know I should be doing. I just keep reaching toward the goal, reminding myself that it is progress, not perfection.

Here are two journal entries that show examples of my processing:

January 5, 1994

Earlier today I pulled out three eyelashes and went into a minor depression. I just returned from a four-mile bike ride, after experiencing a very wet, long winter, and felt the good feelings toward myself that I needed very much today. It gave me relief from the anxiety I was experiencing and a fresh positiveness in my attitude. This gave me the ability to not be pulled into the fear that most often accompanies my pulling episodes. I still had to focus on not touching my lashes, but it provided me with the ability to desire not to pull any more out.

November 22, 1994

Tonight I was able to resist pulling and eating late because I had put so much positive in today. I had the ability to refuse a negative behavior.

Here are some positive verbal affirmations that I have found very helpful, and I hope you will too. These affirmations are offered as a tool to aid in replacing the negative messages of the past with positive messages of recovery.

The remaining material in this chapter is literature from a CoDa meeting I picked up years ago.

JUST FOR TODAY ...

... I will respect myself or my own and others' boundaries.

... I will be vulnerable to someone I trust.

... I will take one compliment and hold it in my heart for more than a fleeting moment. I will let it nurture me.

... I will act in a way that I would admire in someone else.

I am a precious person.

I am beautiful inside and outside.

I love myself unconditionally.

I have ample leisure time without feeling guilty.

I deserve to be loved by myself and by others.

I deserve love, peace, prosperity and serenity.

I forgive myself for hurting myself and others.

I forgive myself for accepting sex when I wanted love.

I forgive myself for letting others hurt me.

I am willing to accept love.

I am not alone, I am loved by God and I belong in this universe.

I am whole and good.

I am capable of changing.

The pain that I might feel by remembering can't be any worse than the pain I feel by knowing and not remembering. Feelings must come before they can go.

I am enough.

(Author unknown, reprinted with permission of AlAnon.)

Here is another piece from my collection:

OUR CIVIL RIGHTS

I have a right to be happy and to be treated with compassion in this home:

> This means that no one will laugh at me or hurt my feelings.

I have the right to be myself in this home:

> This means that no one will treat me unfairly because I am black or white, fat or thin, tall or short, boy or girl, "with hair or without hair" (Author's addition).

I have a right to be safe in this home:

> This means that no one will hit me, kick me, push me, pinch me, or hurt me.

I have a right to hear and be heard in this home:

> This means that no one will yell, scream, rage at me, or shame me.

I have a right to learn about myself in this home:

> This means that I will be free to express my feelings and opinions without being interrupted or punished.

> (Author unknown, reprinted with permission of AlAnon.)

Here is an anonymous piece that I find very helpful in claiming a new outlook.

"RULES FOR BEING HUMAN"

1. **You will receive a body.**

    You may like it or hate it, but it will be yours for the entire period this time around.

2. **You will learn lessons.**

    You are enrolled in a full-time informal school called life. Each day in this school you will have the opportunity to learn lessons. You may like the lessons or think them irrelevant and stupid.

3. **There are no mistakes, only lessons.**

    Growth is a process of trial and error, experimentation. The "failed" experiments are as much a part of the process as the experiment that ultimately "works."

4. **A lesson is repeated until learned.**

    A lesson will be presented to you in various forms until you have learned it. When you have learned it, you can then go to the next lesson.

5. **Learning lessons does not end.**

    There is not part of life that does not contain its lessons. If you are alive, there are lessons to be learned.

6. **"There" is no better than "here."**

    When your "there" has become a "here" you will simply obtain another "there" that will, again, look better than "here."

7. **Others are merely mirrors of you.**

    You cannot love or hate something about another person unless it reflects to you something you love or hate about yourself.

8. **What you make of your life is up to you.**

    You have all the tools and resources you need. What you do with them is up to you. The choice is yours.

9. **Your answers lie inside you.**

    The answers to life's questions lie inside you if you seek with all your heart. All you need to do is look, listen and trust.

    (Cherie Carter-Scott, reprinted with permission of AlAnon.)

I saw this next story on my friend's refrigerator years ago, and copied it, not knowing that I'd ever be putting it in my book.

THE REAL THING

All of us can learn how to be intimate. The first prerequisite is to be intimate with ourselves: to know who we are, what we feel and think, what we want and don't want; and to notice when we are hurt, angry, afraid, lonely, needy, happy or at ease. This means loving someone while staying with yourself and fully participating in your own life rather than escaping on a high. To have a real, intimate relationship, you must be able to:

■ Wait for the relationship to evolve.

■ Be honest when you just don't feel like listening.

■ Care for, rather than take care of, another.

■ Stand by your own values and beliefs, even if they differ from those held by your significant other.

- Realize that your relationship is only one facet of your life.

- Let physical intimacy evolve naturally with emotional intimacy, rather than force or rush it.

- See the other person for what he or she truly is, without judgment.

- Share the other's world while maintaining your own.

- Take risks and be vulnerable.

- Realize that suffering is not love.

- Live your own process and let the other person's unfold on his or her own time schedule.

- Give information freely without trying to control what the other does with it.

- Share your feelings as you experience them.

■ Know that love cannot be created or manipulated, but is a gift that just is.
(Author unknown.)

I want to close this chapter with a poem that I saved from many years ago, when there was only the hope of someday writing this book. It touched my heart and I wanted to share it with you.

I said to the man who stood at the gate of the year,

Give me light that I may tread safely into the unknown—and he replied,

"Go out into the darkness and put your hand into the hand of God,

That shall be to you better than a light and safer than a known way."

(Author unknown.)

6

TRIGGERS FOR PULLING/ RELAXATION TECHNIQUES

Can we change our chemistry by practicing relaxation techniques and eating fewer anxiety-producing foods? Will relaxation techniques change the chemistry in our brain that will lessen the need to pull during anxious times? Is the desire to pull lessened when we eat right, exercise, and release our anxieties to a power greater than ourselves? I believe the answers to these questions is, "Yes!"

How much of our hair pulling is habit and how much is anxiety? I believe by asking these questions we will find answers and by answering these questions we will find relief and release from pulling. I believe it is necessary to be able to identify the different chemicals and anxieties that cause you to pull. My pulling triggers are caffeine, sugar, chocolate, premenstruation, ovulation, stress, feeling overwhelmed, perfectionism, exhaustion and at times the inability to communicate my feelings or take care of myself appropriately.

I believe it is very crucial to identify your feelings. Each time, just do the best you can, and release what you can't identify (believing that it will reveal itself when it's ready). Also, write about what you are feeling, no matter how minimal or trivial it may seem, for there is so much revealed when we put pen to paper. There is much relief to be found when we get it out of ourselves and onto a tangible piece of paper. My best analogy is that it resembles vomiting. When we do not expel the "poison," it just circulates through us repeatedly. Insomnia occurs, stress increases, and confusion grows. Often we will find that what is bothering us is much less than we thought. As we write and discover, then we are peeling the onion and allowing more to be revealed to us. We must take the steps, make the effort, and have courage and be patient, if we want to recover. I believe pulling is only an outward symptom. I believe there is much that needs to be revealed inside us first, before we will stop pulling. One step at a time makes it all possible.

When I first began my journey, my only goal was to have lashes and eyebrows. Today I am so happy at the self-discovery, healing and revelations I have experienced. My priorities have changed and I put less importance on my lack of facial hair. Don't get me wrong, I want so much to go without makeup and not be driven and obsessed with pulling. However, I receive many greater blessings from my lessons than from my hair.

RELAXATION TECHNIQUES & SUGGESTIONS

Breathe in deeply, and tell yourself positive affirmations of truth. As you blow out your air, let out any negative feelings. It amazes me how effective this has been in calming me down.

Listen to relaxation tapes of soothing sounds and muscle relaxation tapes. I have used this technique often, and I usually fall asleep in the process. When I awake it has never failed that I am refreshed and feel like a new person. To my recollection the urges to pull were always lessened. (Be careful of the type of tapes to which you choose to submit your subconscious mind.)

I picked up these next stress managers at a CoDa meeting.

STRESS MANAGEMENT

Things you can do to avoid stress, which will reduce anxiety, thus diffuse the triggers that bring forth the urge to pull:

♦ Get up fifteen minutes earlier.

♦ Prepare for morning the night before.

♦ Don't rely on your memory. Write things down.

♦ Say "no" more often.

♦ Relax unrealistic standards.

♦ Allow for personal time.

♦ Eat nourishing and well-balanced meals, spaced evenly throughout the day.

♦ Get at least seven to eight hours of sleep at night.

PHYSICAL WAYS OF MANAGING STRESS

◆ Sing a favorite song.

◆ Buy clothes that are comfortable and easy to maintain.

◆ Hug your kids, your parents, or a good friend.

◆ Eliminate or restrict the amount of caffeine and alcohol in your diet.

◆ Be good and do good.

◆ Cry.

◆ Laugh.

◆ Take a hot shower or bath.

◆ Do stretching exercises.

◆ Take three deep breaths.

◆ Have a massage.

◆ Listen to your favorite music.

◆ Avoid the company of those who "pull you down."

MENTAL WAYS OF MANAGING STRESS

◆ Accept less-than-perfect performance, but keep working hard to do your best.

◆ Be careful of the "I need it NOW!" mentality.

◆ Remind yourself that you are not responsible for the moods and feelings of others.

◆ Don't pin negative labels on yourself; "I'm so dumb" vs. "Sometimes I do dumb things."

◆ See "failures" as stepping stones instead of roadblocks.

◆ Be willing to learn new things and to unlearn unproductive things.

◆ Accept your "weaknesses" and compensate for them—if you're forgetful, write things down.

◆ Accept your strengths, and use them!

◆ Find the humor in situations.

◆ Change your perspective. Even if our worst fears are realized, they often turn out to be not so bad.

◆ Count your blessings.

◆ Do your best and leave the rest.

◆ Accept your inability to control other people, places and things.

◆ Respect yourself; be your own best friend, not your own worst enemy.

◆ Pray.

◆ Remember you have a choice to laugh or cry; laugh and regain perspective.

◆ Reaffirm your values, ethics and commitment to what is truly important to you.

◆ Don't lower your standards in order to gain the approval of others.

(Author unknown.)

Other techniques for stress reduction and management that I have incorporated into my life are as follows:

Reduce unmanageable jobs to manageable sizes. This can be done by reducing them into mini-jobs. I then cross off each item or job as it is completed and it helps me to keep things simple and clear.

Keep lists. I am big on lists. It helps keep my mind from feeling overwhelmed, because I tend to recount jobs repeatedly in my head so I won't forget what needs to be done. For example, if I'm going to the store I'll write a list of everything I am supposed to get. This way, I don't need to keep my mind unnecessarily occupied. Prioritize your list by numbering what is most important to least important. Sometimes I get overwhelmed thinking that I must complete tasks that truly could wait until another day or time. By looking over my list, arranging the priorities first, it helps me to really appraise the importance or immediacy of each job. Going over this list each morning will organize your day, removing any anxiety from the fear that you might forget an important task, and make your day manageable.

Do not overextend yourself. I used to feel like I had to offer myself when someone would ask for my help or services. I learned to say, "No," without guilt. I recognized that my life and my family's life and well-being were my main priority. This helped me put into perspective what I could and could not do for others. I do offer myself when I am completely able, but I will not sacrifice myself or my family's well-being anymore.

For a long time I said, "No," to many requests. Once I felt better able to function in my own life, I then agreed to extend myself to others' needs. There were times when I initially thought I could fulfill a request, but would then find myself very anxious. I would then have to give myself permission to back out of my commitment after realizing that I had overextended myself. I would try to fulfill an obligation to the best of my ability, but there were a few times I knew I had to apologize and back out. I would always try to make sure that I had given ample warning, to not cause anxiety for another person. Sometimes I was able to fulfill an obligation that I should not have accepted. I would then remind myself to tune in better next time to my situation and needs.

This might sound self-centered to some. The picture I am trying to make clear is the balance of centering on yourself and your needs. I'm not saying you should be selfish and unwilling to give of yourself to others and their needs. Family and self need to come first, or you will have nothing to give others.

As I began to make the effort to get to know myself and my needs, I recognized a need for my own private time. At first it was uncomfortable for me to be alone, going to the beach or to the movies by myself. Eventually, though, it became a cherished time. It was a real necessity, a time for me to reconnect with myself. Only after I have this time with myself to grow and recharge, do I really have anything to offer to my family or others.

7

A PARENT'S STORY

This chapter is to help parents better understand their children's condition. I hope that if you are a parent with a child who pulls, that you will support your child and not chastise them for their pulling behavior. Try to understand what your child is feeling and experiencing. This is why I am opening up my life to you. I hope you will benefit from it, see your child in it, and come to understand them a little bit more.

I was recently speaking to a mother of a puller. She was in such pain to see the beauty of her child disappear as she pulled out her hair, eyelashes and eyebrows. I remembered how I felt when my daughter was lashless and my heart went out to her.

It is a devastating feeling to see the outer beauty of your child leave, because you want the best for them. It is a very terrible, helpless feeling, with which I am very familiar.

I am a mother of children who pull, and am a puller myself. Two of my four children have Trichotillomania. Jessica pulled all her eyelashes out between the ages of five and seven, and now only does it occasionally. Mikaela, who is $4 \, {}^1/_2$ years old, has pulled out her toy bear's fur since she was $1 \, {}^1/_2$.

She has pulled on her eyelashes twice, but has yet to pull any out.

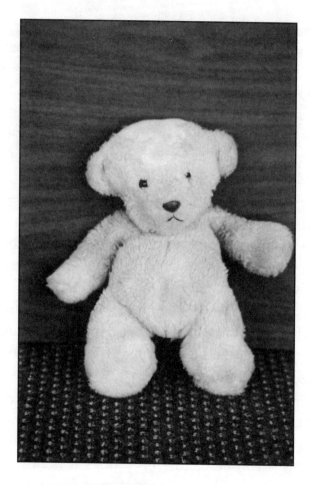

"Bear Bear," Mikaela's favorite toy

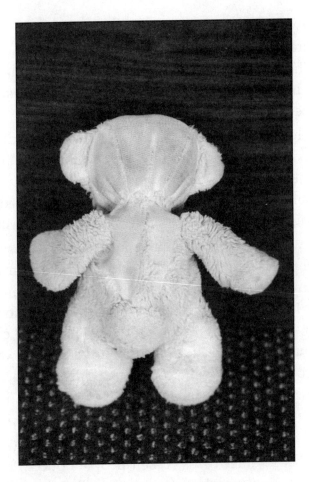

He's missing a third of his fur from
Mikaela pulling it.

I remember the day, as if it were yesterday, when my firstborn, Jessica, walked up to me and I noticed that she had eyelashes missing. There was no question what had happened to them. I knew. My deepest fear had become a reality.

When I was pregnant with each of my children, I prayed for each of them that they would not have to experience Trich. It was the worst thing I could imagine happening to them. Then sure enough, here comes Jessica, five years old, without some of her eyelashes.

It was almost more than I could handle. I was in so much pain when I looked at her because I saw myself and my own suffering, as if she were mirroring me as a child. I felt so much fear for my daughter when I looked at her. I didn't want her to suffer like I had, but I could not imagine it being any easier for her. I definitely wasn't in recovery at that point, so I had no clue. All I had was hate and fear of this behavior. I hated myself, and here was my girl who was gorgeous, who now had pulled out her lashes. They all came out soon after that.

It became her focus. When people noticed, I died inside. I felt like such a failure to myself and to others. I felt that people who noticed that I had no eyelashes would think it was somehow my fault. I felt totally overwhelmed. Jessica still had no eyelashes by the time she entered first grade. She looked different, and I felt

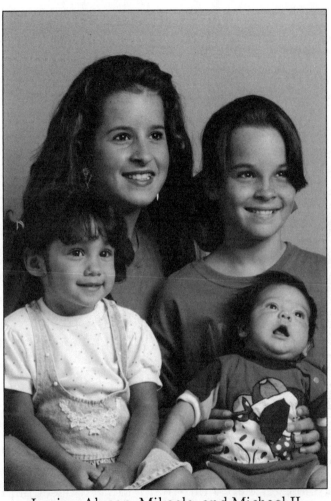

Jessica, Alyson, Mikaela, and Michael II

so embarrassed for her. She had been so beautiful and it was very difficult to see her physical beauty gone now. I also knew that something was going on inside her that I couldn't help. She had always been a very serious little girl. Now it seemed that she was withdrawing inside, just as I had.

Jessica went through her struggles, just as I had feared. Kids would ask her why she had no eyelashes and she'd feel embarrassed. She was definitely affected by it. I told her to come to me any time she wanted to pull, no matter what time of the day or night it was. I suggested she come to me before she pulled, if she could. Many nights, which was when she pulled most, I would hear a knock on my bedroom door and my heart would sink. Fear would run through me, because I knew why she was knocking. Thankfully, most times she had not pulled yet. I would try to help her tune in to what was going on for her, what was prompting her to want to pull. For example, I would ask her if anything was bothering her. She would usually begin by responding that she didn't know. As I would hold her and stroke her face, trying to calm her, she would often begin crying and then get clarity on what had been upsetting her. Sometimes it might be that kids were mean to her at school or that she had pressure from some school assignment. As she would talk about it, her stress would diminish. She'd go back to bed when she felt okay again. The next morning I was always apprehensive to ask her how the night went, and whether she had pulled. To my recollection, she never pulled after our talks.

In second grade she went to a different school and had a wonderful teacher. She was handling it a little better now when kids would ask. In fact, her lashes began to come in, and she'd pull them out less often. It took time, but there definitely was progress.

By the third grade she had them all in. She'd occasionally still pull some, but she definitely didn't pull like she had before.

Over the years she always seems to be missing a few corner lashes, but I am no longer in fear of her pulling all of them out. I know that it is possible that she might struggle more with Trich in her life, but I also know that she has worked recovery in herself. She has developed living skills that help her to cope with life on life's terms. Knowing that she can identify her emotions, I believe that she will less likely need to incorporate pulling into her behavior patterns.

I think it is important for parents to give kids their support, unconditional love and the opportunity to express their stresses and worries. Then they will find that their children's need to pull will lessen as their anxieties decrease.

For the child, and the parent as well, it is important to find some sort of support network. Find someone who understands, such as a therapist or a support group, who can offer help to the child as well as the parent.

I have acceptance for my Trich, and trust for my children's fate. I definitely feel great sadness, though, for the pain they may inevitably have to experience due to Trich. Children's taunts and people's inquiries about their hair, eyelashes or eyebrows always bring so much pain, but the overall picture is what brings hope for myself and my children.

I believe that we who have Trich possess a healthy humility that we'd probably not know if we hadn't had our appearance altered. From that humility comes kindness and recognition of inner value in ourselves and in others.

I am so proud of my daughter. She has faced her Trich with courage and strength. She has taught me many lessons, too, as I have watched her diffuse her perfectionistic tendencies and become more easygoing. Jessica has also helped other child sufferers and shares her story in the following chapter titled, "A Child's Story."

8

A CHILD'S STORY

By Jessica Neve

As a young daughter of a hair puller, I was always intrigued and bewildered by my mother's lack of eyelashes and brows. I had them, but why didn't she? I noticed it but never asked her about it. I was really too young to care much about what went on in other people's lives. I was just beginning to discover and experiment with my own. My understanding was that she just didn't have any. I didn't know she pulled them out. If I had known, I wouldn't have understood why. I had no clue that it was a condition that I would soon be enduring myself; not only a physical pain, but a path of emotional pain and hard learning experiences.

The rest of this story is my own experience with Trichotillomania.

I was probably four or five when I really took notice of my mother's and my own lashes, or rather, my lashes and her lack of them. Mom says that one day I walked up to her and my eyelashes were noticeably thinner. This startled her because of her own pain around her own experiences and her fears since my birth of me ever pulling. She told me that I needed to stop, but I didn't, I couldn't. The next time she saw me, I didn't have any eyelashes. Years later she told me that she was devastated and that she was afraid of the pain I'd have

140

to suffer, as she had. She said every time she'd look at my lashless eyes, she would be reminded of her own pain that she'd experienced as a child. At that time she had not yet begun the process of accepting herself. It would be years before she would begin to find out she was not alone and proceed to heal. But it was not too upsetting to me because I wasn't yet into my looks. It also surprises me that I pulled because I don't recall ever seeing my mom pulling. I felt it was normal for her not to have lashes because that's how I always saw Mom. Well, I continued to pull into elementary school. At first I wasn't at all self-conscious about it, because I wasn't at all concerned with my appearance. I always felt different, feeling like I stuck out in the crowd. I went to a very small private school with about thirty kids in grades one through six. I had several girlfriends. It appeared that my condition of not having lashes didn't bother anyone.

In second and third grade I went to a large Christian private school. Those years became quite traumatic because both my peers and I became very aware of my problem. I guess I had been completely lashless for some time.

But, like Adam and Eve in the Garden of Eden, I wasn't ashamed that I was "naked" until someone pointed it out to me! It was then that I felt I was different. That was when most of the teasing began. I really didn't

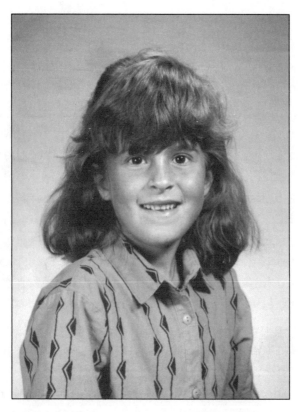

Jessica in the second grade (age seven)

understand why I was singled out. I mean, everyone was different there. Some were too fat, some too skinny. Some were ugly. I was just an average-looking girl who happened to have no eyelashes.

I remember spending quite some time in the bathroom, devastated and crying. I wasn't disliked or an outcast or anything. Maybe teased was not the right word, but all the kids (including my friends) would ask me questions like, "Where are your eyelashes?" and say things like, "That's weird." I got so self-conscious about it that my mom tried to help me by putting eyeliner on me. Unfortunately, it was very noticeable. It just brought me more unwanted attention, sometimes even by my teachers. I decided not to wear it anymore.

Those two years are what I believe kind of pushed me into putting up a wall, a type of protective shell. I was far from shy, but I tended to overly care what other people thought of me. I never felt like I fit in around people. After third grade I was very happy to leave that school. I believe it was during that summer that I was able to let my lashes grow back, but it still really hurt. I remember when a friend who had eczema on her eyelids asked me about mine. She didn't say it rudely or teasingly. She just asked, but I took it the wrong way and I started to cry. It hurt whenever someone pointed it out to me.

At the beginning of fourth grade I still felt scared, awkward and very self-conscious about myself, even though my eyes were now full of lashes. It was my first public school and I didn't know anyone there. New situations always made me uncomfortable.

The next two years, little did I know, would be the best and worst two years of my whole life. From the get-go I knew that I absolutely did not fit in with this group of snobby, rich, stuck-up kids who had all known each other since around kindergarten. And I didn't want to fit in, probably because I knew I couldn't. To make things worse, I was also quite a tacky dresser. (My mom didn't realize that fashion even mattered at that age, and my parents didn't have much money, either.) I don't think my not fitting in had much to do with my personality. More that, though, I was withdrawn from the pain I had gone through in the previous years. Well, no matter how horrible I remember those years to be, I will always remember the day I first met Heather, my best friend.

I sat in the front of my fourth grade classroom. The teacher greeted everyone in the class and then said, "I see we have a set of twins in this class." Well, everyone else knew who they were, but I looked carefully around and spotted two identical girls. I soon bonded with one of them, and we became the best of friends. My only really good memories of those two years were with Heather. Best of all, she knew about my pulling problem and she didn't care. She made me feel like I was her sister. We have become incredibly close since then, but at that time in my life things were going incredibly wrong. My parents split after a ten-year marriage and I went through a really painful period in my life. Heather was there for me through my parents' divorce. A few years later my mom remarried and gave me and my sister, Alyson, a new little sister and brother. That was when things really changed. My mom and my new stepdad decided to move my family away from my home in Santa Cruz, California. I had been born and raised there for nine years. I had to leave my best friend and my father to move to Sacramento, California, a city I had never been to and where I knew no one. That was when the pulling kicked in again.

In sixth grade I began to pull again, although it wasn't enough for people to notice. There were often thin areas or bare patches. I was still withdrawn and again did not fit in with my peers. We didn't stay in Sacramento for much more than a year because my stepdad's job moved us to Fremont, California. We stayed there for three months and then moved back to Sacramento by the beginning of seventh grade. Junior high was exciting for me. It was not always easy, but it was exciting. I got into a lot of trouble. I joined the wrong crowds and learned a lot from the mistakes I made, but I loved school (though my grades didn't reflect it!) and my friends. I also had lots of freedom, of which I often took full advantage. My dad moved up from Santa Cruz with his fiance and her two kids at the end of eighth grade. Well, junior high ended and due to my grades I had to go to summer school. I got into trouble there, too. I dyed my hair purple and pierced my own belly button. So my parents decided to send me to a private school again. I was crushed. I wanted to be with my friends. My pulling was getting more noticeable and I had many bare patches. The school was very small, but I liked it. My pulling didn't bother me much until a friend asked me one day in P.E. why I had eyelashes missing. I told her it was because I wore too much mascara and my eyelashes got brittle, so when I played with or pulled on my mascara, my lashes fell out. Well, it was partly the truth! Then my dad and his fiance, Tina, decided to move to Redding, California. That was tough.

Just last semester my parents pulled me out of that school because my grades never went up. They decided to home-school me. It ended up helping me a lot because it took a lot of the pressure out my life.

At that point I started wanting to go to church on my own. I have been going to a great church for a year now. My self-confidence is strong and I love myself a lot. My pulling is coming under control for the most part. It still can be a daily fight, but not always. At the moment I am missing half of each set of lower lashes, but I'll probably have them in and out for the next few months or more, if not for the rest of my life. My life is just beginning and I'm excited about my future. By the grace of God, my pulling is becoming manageable. I am only fifteen years old and I know that this will most likely be a lifelong struggle. The worst is over, though, because I don't pull as much anymore. Praise God! Through all this time my mom and I have bonded through our pulling and are very close friends. She has helped me when I've needed her or wanted to pull. At those times when she's been pulling and needing support, I have tried to help her, too. She's always there for me, even in the middle of the night when I have needed someone to hold me, to pray for me, and to help me identify what is really bothering me. This has always worked for me. I couldn't have done it without her.

Sometimes I'll just start pulling and I'm not even aware of it. My hands will just go to my eyes whenever I am stressed or mad or excited or anything. I really have to make myself stop and think about what I am doing. I have to realize that if I don't stop I will be lashless by morning. If that doesn't help, then I sit on my hands, read a book, write, or do anything that I can to distract myself and make myself stop. Exercise helps a lot. I've always managed to stop pulling before they're all gone. Sometimes I wish that I could just pull them all out instead of dealing with the feelings of restlessness and anxiety. Then I could just stay in my house until they all grew back, but of course that's not realistic. I don't want to isolate myself anymore. So I just tell myself that if I don't pull I will look better physically and feel much better about myself emotionally. Sometimes, though, I don't even have the desire to stop pulling.

Today I am happy and confident. I've discovered my inner beauty and it shows. It feels good when many people who used to exclude me notice me and now seek my friendship. I've really changed for the better through my whole experience, and I hope you discover your inner beauty, too.

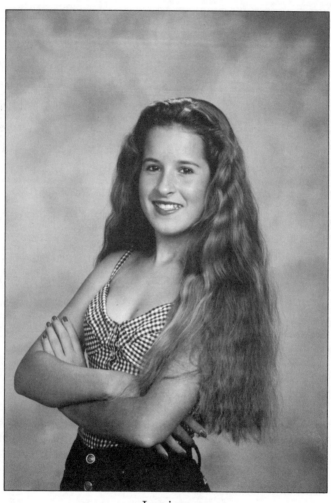

Jessica
(age fifteen)

9

A MATE'S STORY

by Michael Salazar

For this chapter I chose to do an interview with my husband. I hope it helps other mates of people who pull.

I really respect Mike's outlook. Mike is a person who is willing to look at his own "stuff." He has always given me the freedom to be an individual. I feel very safe in his presence, naked with no makeup as well as with makeup on. He has always treated me as beautiful. It has taken me a long time to be able to receive it and believe it, to feel attractive and sexual (because I pull my pubic hair), but his attitude has been such a healing tool for me. Now I have been really able to accept it and embrace it.

Mike is one who has worked very hard on his life. He has not always been such a wise, good person. We have worked a lot in our marriage to come to a place where we don't point fingers at each other, but we each look at our own life. So he really is speaking from a place of having worked what he's talking about. I have such a high respect for him.

It is very important to have a husband's perspective, because I have heard of many husbands who really give their wives who pull a hard time, shaming them or treating them disrespectfully. Perhaps if they can hear from another person who is a mate of a puller, it can encourage them to gain a new perspective. The person who pulls also can see that they don't deserve to be treated in a disrespectful way. Sometimes when we are only around one adult in our life and they are unsafe and unsupportive, we can think that everybody would be like that. We think, "I must deserve this, because this is my mate and they love me more than anyone." So here is another perspective. They can realize that no, it is not normal or appropriate to have anyone judging and criticizing them for pulling or any other situation or flaw in their beauty.

Mike began with an offer to other mates:

Mike: I would be willing to talk to any mate of a puller or non-puller just to let them know what I go through and how I feel. It is not always easy. I'm not always able to look past myself enough to love her and help her because I go through my own feelings. I get angry because she's lashing out at me. The whole thing is that we need to recognize it. Once it is recognized, then it can be addressed.

Cheryn: At the beginning of our dating, about a month into our relationship, I remember when I first pulled my eyelashes enough that I was afraid to see you. I called you and said that I had pulled my eyelashes. What did you feel the first time I told you that I had pulled out my eyclashes and that I had Trichotillomania?

Mike: My feelings have always been more concern about you than about me. I always just wanted to comfort you and let you know that it doesn't matter to me. I've never, ever had any emotions around your pulling. The only reaction that I have ever had is basically that when you pull, it affects me by how you react. The only emotion your pulling has ever done to me, outside of the effect of your emotions, is just that I want to reassure you and comfort you, letting you know that it doesn't matter to me. I love you either way, whether you have them or whether you don't, because it really doesn't matter.

Cheryn: But outside that, my mood changes.

Mike: Well, that is where it gets hard, because you pull away. At times you react toward me or the kids; angry, sad. You put walls up. I can't tell you what feelings you're feeling, I can only tell what your reactions are to your feelings. It gets really emotional.

Cheryn: When you first found out I pulled, did you have any emotions around it?

Mike: No, because I've been in recovery. I know we all have our ways of coping. This was just your way of coping, whatever the case may be.

Cheryn: Had you ever heard of Trichotillomania before? Didn't it seem odd?

Mike: No. No.

Cheryn: So when I first showed you my eyes after telling you on the phone that I had pulled, what happened after I drove up to you?

Mike: I said, "Okay, let's get this over with." Knowing you felt uncomfortable, I wanted to reassure you so I looked at them and said, "They look fine to me."

Cheryn: I remember you kissed my eyes and then gave me a hug.

Mike: I always try to do that just for the fact that obviously you are hurting. Sometimes when you pull, you won't let me near you emotionally. You'll pull, and you'll use different ways without saying, "Get away from me." You'll be angry about a certain thing, something would be magnified around the house. Your emotions will be magnified, so if I were to do something you would get hurt really easily. I might do something that may be a normal thing that happens every day and it just caught you at a time you were pulling and you were sensitive to it. That's where it really gets hard for me.

Cheryn: How many days, after I have pulled, do my emotions stay this way?

Mike: I'm not sure. I know it has lessened each time you pull, since you have accepted it and been willing to grow through it.

Cheryn: Has it gotten any better?

Mike: Yes. Also because you have grown, you seem to notice when you are in that place so it gives you serenity to know it will pass.

Cheryn: Would you notice a depression?

Mike: I don't think there was any one standard pattern outside of the fact that your emotions would be exaggerated, and you would be more sensitive, pessimistic.

Cheryn: How did you feel when my lashes and brows would be coming in?

Mike: Again, to be completely honest, I don't notice it. I don't notice when they are coming in, and I don't notice when they are out. All I know is by what you tell me, or every now and then I'll notice that your eyelashes are in.

Cheryn: Does it look more attractive to you?

Mike: You couldn't be any more beautiful to me, bald or not. The only thing that is less attractive about this whole thing is how you act after you've pulled. That's the only thing that is less attractive.

Cheryn: So it wouldn't bother you if I had half of my hair missing?

Mike: No. Could you ever feel that it didn't matter to me? How does that make you feel that I don't care?

Cheryn: Very wonderful. I don't feel like you are examining me.

Mike: But have you always felt that? Do you feel that way when you are in the middle of it? Do you feel like I am watching you?

Cheryn: No, not anymore. I never felt that you were thinking, "Ew." But I always wondered if you were thinking anything. How about your fear when you see Mikaela pulling on her bear's hair?

Mike: That makes me a little nervous. It's not the look that bothers me, but the concern for what's going on inside. That's always been my focus and my attention and my care giving. It's not the pulling, the action, but what is going on underneath that's making you or her want to do that.

Cheryn: What if she pulled out all of her hair, what would you feel?

Mike: I'd feel sad for her. Because if she does that, she obviously has something going on.

Cheryn: Would you feel angry toward me for passing on these genetics of Trichotillomania?

Mike: I can't say that I would. I would like to think that I wouldn't blame or be angry with you. I know I would feel for her, seeing what you go through and knowing that she'd have to experience something along that line.

Cheryn: I know I would feel very sad knowing that in this world of superficial values, that she'd be ostracized. She would look different, and she wouldn't have her beauty. So what would you say to the men out there who criticize their wives?

Mike: Don't. I mean, look at yourself before you look at anybody else. We all have our problems. We are not perfect, and it's not fair for anyone to do that. The only advice I'd ever give anybody is to try and love them through it and let them know that they're loved, period. That's all that has to happen and that's all we can do. We can't change them. We can't do anything but let them know that we love them anyway. If we can't do that, then we need to get help around it, because it is not our problem. We need to learn how to deal with it, in a way that is not destructive to the person that's pulling.

Cheryn: I have heard many husbands say that they are irritated by it, or they are repulsed by it.

Mike: I think that's their own insecurities. Why should how their mate looks matter to them? How many of those men have potbellies? How many of those men sit on the couch and drink beer? How many of those men don't take care of their wives the way they should? How many don't love themselves?

Cheryn: What do you say to the men who do keep their bodies in shape and do have discipline?

Mike: I don't care what they are doing. They have no right to judge anyone else. The worst thing they can do for somebody is to put more emotion and weight on that person. Then the mate who is pulling has to carry the anxiety that the husband is feeling.

Anyone who is pulling has their own stuff that they have to carry. Why should they have to carry their mate's, too? Focusing on their mate in the first place indicates something is wrong within themselves and out of balance in their life.

Cheryn: It sounds to me like a control issue. What do you think about anyone who is trying to control someone?

Mike: Well, that is a dysfunction in itself. We all try to do the best we can with how to live life, with the tools that we do or don't have. It is not any more fair for me to control you than for you to control me. I know I don't like it if I'm asked, "Where'd you go? What have you been doing? Why did you do that?" Nobody wants to hear that. What right does anyone have to do that? So what right would I have to say, "It really bothers me when you pull," or, "I wish you'd grow some eyelashes." It is not fair to any human being to do that. I don't believe that's how God intends a mate to be.

Cheryn: What is your concept of marriage? What should a marriage partnership be?

Mike: More than the standard fifty-fifty, and give. What I have learned, now that I have God in my life, is it is all about being a servant. I need to serve you and my children. Period. Can I do it? No, not all the time. I am just as self-centered as probably anybody can be. I have my moments when I'm better than at other times. Since I have entered recovery, and have God in my life, it is getting better with time. But it's just like the Bible says, be a servant and put someone else's needs before your own. That's what I believe a marriage is to be about.

Cheryn: What would that say about a mate who was embarrassed by their mate's appearance?

Mike: That would say that they're too engrossed in their mate. I need to be my own individual and let you be your own individual. I need to get my own self-esteem. I'm not going to get it from you. I should never feel that you are my possession. What you are and what you do should not reflect how I feel about myself. Nobody should ever feel that way.

Cheryn: Why do you think people ever feel that their mate's appearance is a reflection of them?

Mike: They are getting their self-esteem from the wrong place. There is not one person or one thing outside of ourselves and our relationship to God that is going to make us feel whole.

That's probably what happens when they get engrossed in the mate's pulling. You think you have problems with their appearance? Climb inside. Be the puller for a while. See what that feels like. I know I wouldn't want to walk in her shoes.

Cheryn: I know when Jessica pulled, when she was a little girl, it embarrassed me when people would see her. Since I hadn't yet worked on my self-esteem, I would feel that she reflected my inadequacies as a mother, especially if they noticed I had missing brows or lashes. I also had incredible guilt and anxiety about her pulling.

There are many times a parent will spank or punish a child when they see that the child has been pulling. What would your comment be on that?

Mike: Don't. They are doing it for a reason. It is a defense mechanism, either a way to shut down or a way of self-abuse. They are no different from someone who may be abusing drugs or alcohol, compulsively washing their hands, or biting their fingernails. We have come a long way and there is a lot of help out there and awareness for us. We realize, now, that we do things for a reason. We are all, no matter who, from the most abusive person to the nicest person, we are all dysfunctional because we are human. We all do things, and we're all just trying to do the best we can with the tools we have to live life. Whether it is a child or an adult, their pulling is for some reason. It's their way of coping. That's what it is all about. It needs to be recognized that way, because those of us who don't pull want to be loved through our faults, physical or not. Nobody is faultless.

Cheryn: Thank you very much for this interview.

Mike: You're welcome.

MY POEM TO MICHAEL

How blessed has been the help of my husband, Michael.

He has been one to hold out his hand to hold mine,

His hand assisting me up the stairs, one step at a time.

My other hand is held by God, who also carries my foot in His palm

So when I feel afraid to move forward,

He helps me to lift my foot a little higher.

© 1995 Cheryn Salazar

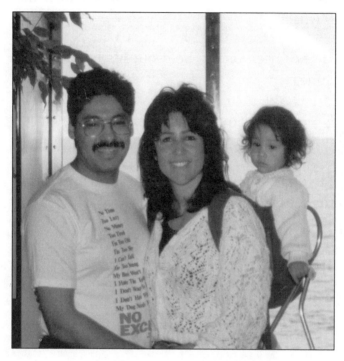

Michael, Cheryn, and Mikaela

❧ 10 ❧

RECOVERY

Several years ago I became aware that I needed to make some changes in my life, to do some major emotional growing. I recognized that I was dysfunctional in how I perceived and handled certain issues in my life. I've never been one to adapt to changes easily, and I was very apprehensive of what this would entail. While attending an Alcoholics Anonymous twelve-step group I read a definition of recovery that brought me a lot of peace and a feeling of great relief because I tend to be very impatient with myself. It said, "Recovery is not a place of destination, but a road on which you travel." (Author unknown.)

My own definition is, "Recovery is the discovery and healing of areas in your being that had not been given the correct environment or information to mature in the way intended." For me, it has meant learning to feel my feelings, to trust and respect myself, to recognize that I am a valuable person, to set boundaries to protect myself from unsafe people or situations, and to respect and trust my own process as I walk on this road of recovery.

For me it was imperative to remove the voice of perfectionism that told me that I wasn't arriving fast enough, and to also know that it would be a life journey and that no one achieves perfection. I just needed to do my best. I felt much comfort in this.

My pace and process of recovery unfolded for me exactly as it needed to, and in its own perfect timing.

I believe that we were all made to walk some road of recovery. Trials teach us many things, and until our life is over, I don't think our "road" will ever end. I also truly believe that we were meant to live a life of quality. If we don't possess that outlook, we will be bitter about our trials. We will miss out on all the lessons that life offers to teach us.

Trichotillomania can cause you to look harder to find true contentment, peace and happiness. When you have to look harder, it makes you look deeper. You benefit by discovering a treasure you might have never discovered before.

From the look of our society as a whole, I believe this path is certainly the road less traveled.

When I recognized that society has a very distorted value system in our world, basing our worth on our outward appearance, I began to recognize how dysfunctional our society is. I realized that I didn't have to "buy into it" anymore.

I began to venture out on my own to define a correct evaluation of life. I found it very interesting that just a century ago, being thin and tan was very unfashionable. It meant that you were poor and hungry and worked in a field. Being twenty to forty pounds overweight and pale meant that you were wealthy. I became completely convinced that I no longer had to feel like I wasn't okay if I didn't fit into the trends of our society.

I have always recognized a great pain in those who feel they don't fit into society's measurement of worth. I believe we are the pioneers, the people of our generation who have challenged our society's stereotypes, recognizing its fallacies and destructiveness.

The following analogy describes my journey on this road.

I have found the road of recovery has many diverse topographies There are mountains to climb, some steeper than others, and there are valleys to coast down, which offer a breather. The rocks may cause us to stumble, but a stumble might prevent us from a fall! Storms may soak us through and thunder might startle us, but the day afterward the air will be cleaner and clearer. Hailstones will force us to move from discomfort to search for safe places of protection.

The lessons I have learned from this journey have taught me so much more than I ever could have imagined. Today I am a stronger person who enjoys life. My lack of hair does not hinder me in my participation of life anymore. I hope you come to a place where you are able to embrace life in its fullest, too.

I believe trials are in our life to teach us to grow. I also truly believe that we were meant to live a life of quality, to be able to overcome every difficulty we encounter. The tools are within us and it takes courage to find them. The most valuable lessons I've learned have come through my most difficult circumstances.

I believe we must expose and feel our pain in order to heal. The help of someone outside yourself, who is safe and nonjudgmental, is necessary for us to process our pain effectively.

Honesty begets honesty in our own self, and if we can be around someone that we trust, then we can open up and share about ourselves. This gives us the ability to learn to trust ourselves. It can help give us the courage and the insight to not respond to ourselves negatively.

As I mentioned before, the support group I attend has been a great help toward my recovery. Knowing that I am not alone is such a relief. I have been attending support groups for several years and they have helped me grow in many different dimensions. When I began attending the Trichotillomania support meetings I believe my self-esteem began to heal and grow. I had previously begun to work on accepting and loving myself unconditionally, but to actually be surrounded by fellow pullers helped me identify my experiences with their own stories. This really let my soul know I was not strange, weird, or any other devastating label I had been given or had given myself in my life. I am still amazed to hear the familiar tales being told at meetings by fellow hair pullers. They all have felt my pain. Many have experienced the same discomforts as I, such as fear of my makeup coming off if I swam, cried, perspired or rubbed my eyes, and going to the beautician, to name only a few.

In my life I have spent many hours pulling, much time feeling isolated as if I were a freak, much time in sheer panic, fearing someone might notice and mention my "abnormality." Today I have a confidence because I finally know that I am not strange. I no longer value my self-worth by my appearance, therefore I no longer feel shame if people notice that I have no eyelashes or eyebrows. However, I do look forward to the day when I can go without makeup for the freedom of it, and I believe with all my heart that it will be in the near future.

I am finding that as I go to meetings I learn more about myself and what triggers my pulling episodes. There is something so spiritual that happens deep inside me and I see the fruits of the support group in my life today. I also see changes happening to the others in my group.

To all fellow Trichotillomania sufferers, I'd like to say: I am very hopeful for you, even if you are not. There is so much to be revealed. I believe that you will find so much more than success over pulling: a deeper knowledge and a new love for yourself. You now know that you are not alone. I know that when I found out there were others who pulled I began to feel less alone and a multifaceted healing process began in my life. I believe with all of my heart that this same freedom is available to you, too.

Since I knew of no one else that pulled, my journey has been a long and painful road. There were no road maps given to me. I didn't know there were others who had gone before me, reaching places of peace with their condition (in some cases, complete remission from pulling). If I had known I wasn't alone, I surely would have had an easier time. This is my desire and my reason for writing this book. I am happy to be alive and the misery is gone. I know that if I had heard someone say this, it would have given me a hope for my life.

Because the pain goes so deep and affects, in most cases, our entire being, we need to come out of isolation.

We tend to be master isolators. By having someone to talk to, we begin to draw out of ourselves the issues that contribute to our pulling and our negative self-esteem. Talking lets the shame be released. I truly believe that everyone has something with which to contend. This helped me to accept that Trichotillomania was my "something" and that I did indeed fit into the norm of society. I always would have preferred to be a nail-biter instead, but I now have accepted that this is my lot in life.

Pain can either cause you to emotionally shut down or emotionally open up and grow. I chose, and continue to choose to open up and grow. We must expose and feel pain in order to heal.

My heart feels the pain of my family of pullers, the estimated six to eight million of us. I am looking forward to the day when I feel the joy and release from the pulling urge more on a daily basis. I believe that can happen. I have already experienced it for a time. The pulling is becoming less frequent, and the duration between pulling is lengthening. There are many who share my testimony of recovery from pulling and recovery from the damage that Trichotillomania had inflicted upon their life. This can be your experience, too, if you are willing to walk the road—your road of recovery.

The following, "Letting Go," is one of the tools that helped me function better in my life. I hope it will help you, too.

LETTING GO

These are instructions on how to let go. Perhaps it is of a rebellious child or a burden of sorrow, losing a loved one or learning to live with a heartache which you just cannot let go of. Read this over, study it, pray over it, and you will find that which will allow your spirit to soar—to be free, to completely give it all to God—and let the work be done within you, where the need is.

- To let go doesn't mean to stop caring, it means I can't do it for someone else.

- To let go is not to cut myself off, it is the realization that I can't control another.

- To let go is not to enable, but to allow learning from natural consequences.

- To let go is not to try to change or blame another, I can only change myself.

- To let go is to admit powerlessness, which means the outcome is not in my hands.

- To let go is not to care for, but to care about.

- To let go is not to fix, but to be supportive.

- To let go is not to judge, but to allow another to be a human being.

- To let go is not to be in the middle, arranging outcomes, but to allow others to effect their own outcomes.

- To let go is not to be protective, it is to permit another to face reality.

- To let go is not to deny, but to accept.

- To let go is not to nag, scold or argue, but to search out my own shortcomings and then correct them.

- To let go is not to adjust everything to my desires, but to take each day as it comes and to cherish the moment.

- To let go is not to criticize and regulate anyone, but to try to become what I dream I can be.

- To let go is not to regret the past, but to grow and live in serenity and peace.

- To let go is to fear less and love more.

  (Author unknown, reprinted by permission of AlAnon.)

There is a wonderful inner peace that we attain when we discover the truth of our own worth. The following is from an article describing some signs and symptoms of inner peace. These signs and symptoms are:

- A tendency to think and act spontaneously rather than on fears based on past experiences.

- An unmistakable ability to enjoy each moment.

- A loss of interest in judging other people.

- A loss of interest in judging self.

- A loss of interest in interpreting the actions of others.

- A loss of interest in conflict.

- A loss of the ability to worry.

- Frequent, overwhelming episodes of appreciation.

- Contented feelings of connectedness with others and nature.

- Frequent attacks of smiling.

- An increasing tendency to let things happen rather than make them happen.

- An increased susceptibility to the love extended by others as well as the uncontrollable urge to extend it.

(Author unknown.)

Freedom from obsessive behaviors comes from true surrender. True surrender isn't when we are having to "white knuckle" it.

When the urge to pull or overeat overcomes me, I ask myself questions like, "What is it that I am really wanting right now? Is it an emotional need? Do I want attention, love, or am I feeling angry or sad and I don't know how to handle it?" When we begin to realize what it is that makes us want to act out, addressing the situation from the inside out, then we find freedom. We then begin to get our answers.

If I am just trying to "white knuckle" or control the addiction and the behavior, then I end up struggling. That is not recovery. I might very well stop the behavior physically, but if I have not dealt with the root of the problem, it will just manifest itself in another negative behavior. This is like the alcoholic who stops drinking but never changes the behavior. They are often referred to as "dry drunks." People can also transfer their addiction to smoking, overeating, sexual addiction, etc.

Emotional development is recovery. When we learn to address the real issues which preceded the dysfunctional behaviors, then we change and become whole, and our life recovers.

I recognize today that my hair pulling has been just as much a drug to me as alcohol and overeating have been. Pulling gives me the same type of release from stress.

I have found that the twelve steps adapted from Alcoholics Anonymous helped me to learn living skills so I could live a new way. (I am now seven years sober.) These skills helped me to learn to know myself better and to identify and express my feelings appropriately. They have proven themselves to be very effective for people with Trichotillomania who incorporate them into their lives. The steps were developed originally in AA. They teach people living skills and how to identify their feelings instead of shutting down emotionally by using vices or acting out inappropriately.

I am not saying that all pulling is due to shutting down emotionally. What I am saying is that this is one major reason in my life and with most of the pullers that I have personally contacted.

These steps offer a number of skills that teach you how to be honest with yourself and others, to live in a way that promotes healthy emotional and physical behaviors. By using these skills, our need to zone out or be numb becomes unnecessary. For this reason I am including them at the end of this chapter. I highly encourage you to find a support group of some kind that possesses this kind of format for recovery. These steps offer life skills to help you function on life's terms. Working the steps will help you with issues that promote behaviors which are manifest in negative ways. I encourage you to check for yourself to see which scenarios apply to you.

Here are the twelve steps of Alcoholics Anonymous. A space appears in place of the word "alcohol" in Step 1 and "alcoholics" in step 12.

AN ADAPTATION OF THE TWELVE STEPS

1. We admitted we were powerless over _____, and that our lives had become unmanageable.

2. Came to believe that a Power greater than ourselves could restore us to sanity.

3. Made a decision to turn our will and our lives over to the care of God as we understood Him.

4. Made a searching and fearless moral inventory of ourselves.

5. Admitted to God, to ourselves, and to another human being the exact nature of our wrongs.

6. Were entirely ready to have God remove all these defects of character.

7. Humbly asked God to remove our shortcomings.

8. Made a list of all persons we had harmed, and became willing to make amends to them all.

9. Made direct amends to such people whenever possible, except when to do so would injure them or others.

10. Continued to take personal inventory and when we were wrong promptly admitted it.

11. Sought through prayer and meditation to improve our conscious contact with God as we understood Him, praying only for knowledge of God's will for us and the power to carry that out.

12. Having had a spiritual awakening as a result of these steps, we tried to carry this message to _____ and to practice these principles in all our affairs.

THE TWELVE STEPS OF
ALCOHOLICS ANONYMOUS

1. We admitted we were powerless over alcohol, and that our lives had become unmanageable. 2. Came to believe that a Power greater than ourselves could restore us to sanity. 3. Made a decision to turn our will and our lives over to the care of God as we understood Him. 4. Made a searching and fearless moral inventory of ourselves. 5. Admitted to God, to ourselves, and to another human being the exact nature of our wrongs. 6. Were entirely ready to have God remove all these defects of character. 7. Humbly asked God to remove our shortcomings. 8. Made a list of all persons we had harmed, and became willing to make amends to them all. 9. Made direct amends to such people whenever possible, except when to do so would injure them or others. 10. Continued to take personal inventory and when we were wrong promptly admitted it. 11. Sought through prayer and meditation to improve our conscious contact with God as we understood Him, praying only for knowledge of God's will for us and the power to carry that out. 12. Having had a spiritual awakening as a result of these steps, we tried to carry this message to alcoholics and to practice these principles in all our affairs.

The following five steps were adapted for Trichotillomania Support Groups by Carol Anderson, with permission from AA.

FIVE STEPS OF TA

1. **Surrender**

   We recognize and accept that we are powerless to stop our hair pulling. We surrender absolutely.

2. **Commitment**

   We seek support and spiritual enrichment through group process. By sharing our dilemma we learn to reach outside ourselves for help and guidance.

3. **Willingness**

   Our commitment to recovery from hair pulling is expressed in our willingness to help and be helped through all available means of recovery. There are no bounds to our willingness for this is the door to spiritual freedom.

4. **Shame Reduction**

   We believe that hair pulling does not have to be a shame-oriented disorder. Through group process, we hope to reduce our shame and in so doing open the doors to self-esteem. Self-esteem is the courage to recover.

5. **Recovery**

Building our self-esteem is the heartbeat of our program. Through this process we improve our relationships with each other, with ourselves, and with the world. By helping ourselves we learn to help others and through helping others we recover.

I began my first step in self-help by dealing with my overeating. I read a book called Feeding the Hungry Heart by Geneen Roth. She mentioned that she had quit dieting and forbidding herself food. At first she gained a lot of weight and then her body began to drop that weight and more until her body reached a weight at which it was comfortable. She also had to learn not to feed her body when it was not hungry, as she previously would feed herself when she would be stressed or emotional.

First I gave myself permission to eat whatever I wanted. I received the benefits that she had spoken of and decided to apply this approach to my hair pulling. I gave myself permission to pull for a year, whenever I needed, respecting that it was a way I nurtured and took care of myself at that time in my life. I wanted to begin loving myself. I knew I had to remove the negative emotions that I had attached to pulling in the past in order to heal myself from all the emotional pain Trich had brought to me. By doing this, I was giving up all the hatred I had attached to myself and my Trich.

I also gave up the dream that I'd never pull again. This goal had actually been the contributor to much disappointment and depression, both of which had been very damaging. I still hope to someday quit pulling, but even if I don't stop, I am now able to accept myself regardless of the outcome. It took away the pressure and freed me up to start learning to love and accept myself. I put less power in my hairs. Sure enough, there was a point after about a year that I began to desire not to pull. It wasn't because I had to stop or should stop, but because I wanted to stop.

The same thing happened with the food. It was like having cake in my house all the time. The temptation left because I knew I could have it any time I wanted. Allowing myself to pull let go of the guilt, pressure and the overwhelmed feelings that previously always followed, which usually spiraled me into more self-destructive behavior.

My life has gained better perspective and balance since I am no longer focusing on my hair as much. I want this for you, too. I have a few questions that I want to propose to you which I have also asked myself.

Where will you be in ten years? Will you be the same emotionally, different only in appearance, or will you have decided to change and grow emotionally?

My goal is to take care of myself emotionally and physically. Change is difficult, but not changing is harder in the long run. I have experienced tremendous fear and anxiety when recognizing certain areas in my life that needed change, but it is through surrendering to God that I have received peace.

When I finally realized that I was unable to change these things by myself and that others had found help when they handed their addictions or compulsions over to a "Higher Power," I tried it myself. That was when I truly found the answers and the solutions. My life began to change.

My recovery process has included seven years of pain, struggle and sadness. It has gotten easier over time, but it has been no easy road.

This process of recovery is like having a baby. It takes a long time. After the seed is planted, it takes time to develop. Your body changes and finally one day you give birth. After all the pain and discomfort, the hormonal changes and the delivery, you end up with the gift of a beautiful baby. I really like what has come forth from my experience with Trichotillomania. It has been at great cost, but well worth it.

I imagine once I finish this book I'll think of many more things I'd have liked to include in this chapter. I hope that you have been able to get to know me and hopefully identify yourself with me, so that you will no longer feel alone.

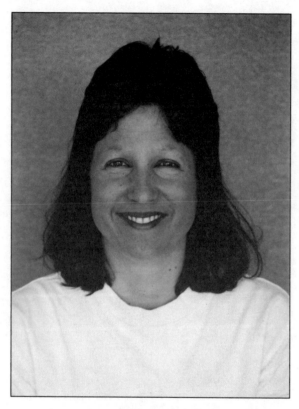

Before makeup

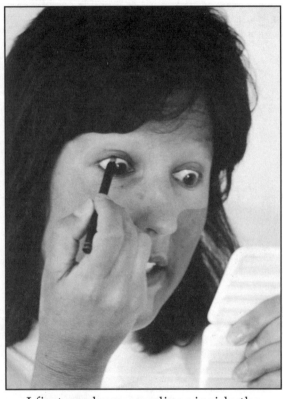

I first apply my eyeliner inside the
upper lid where lashes would
normally grow.

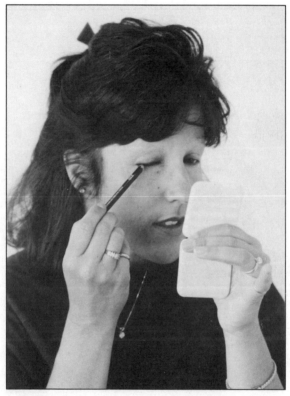

I then lightly draw in where eyeliner
would normally be applied. This gives the
appearance of eyelashes.

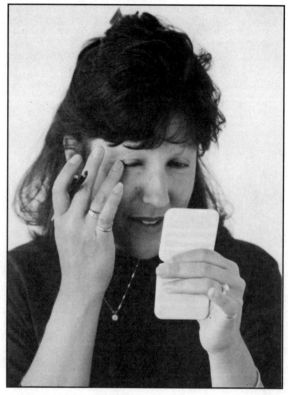

I lightly smudge makeup to give it a
softer look.

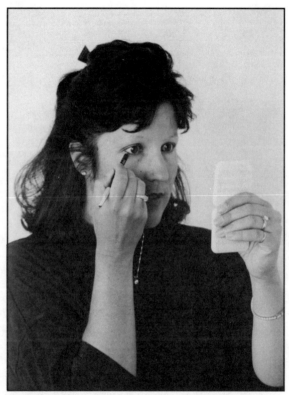

I apply lower lid eyeliner the same way.

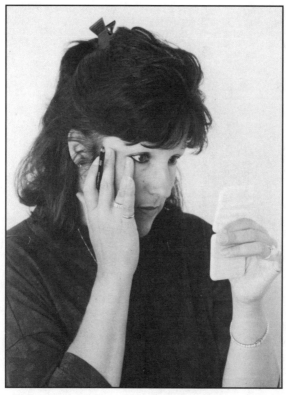

Then I smudge it, too, for a softer look.

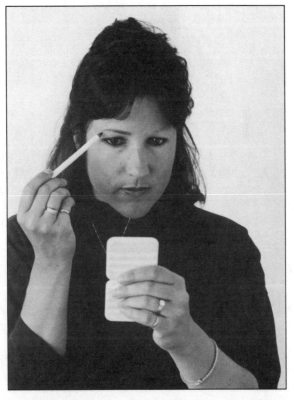

I begin drawing my eyebrows in with
light strokes, repeating until dark enough.
I try to create a look that resembles eyebrows
as best I can. Remember, light, soft strokes.

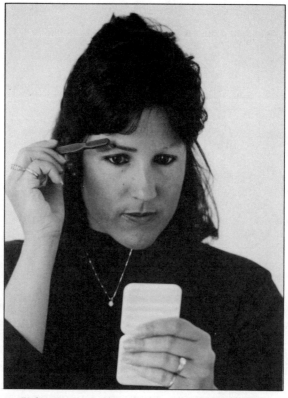

I then use a brush (a soft toothbrush
works fine) to lightly blend any uneven
areas. I don't want the eyebrow to look
hand-drawn.

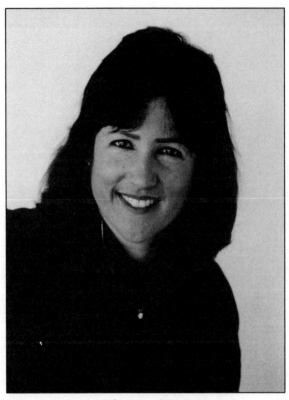

After makeup

11

JOURNAL ENTRIES
&
POETRY CLIPS

Journal writing helps us to identify our own feelings and emotions. There truly is "power in the pen." I've heard that phrase all of my life, but I never understood until I tried it. I encourage you to try it. If this overwhelms you, maybe you could begin by talking into a tape recorder. I found that to be very simple. The benefit is that it helps you to get out of your head. Whatever catalyst you use, remember to "be gentle" with yourself. This was what Christina Pearson, (the founder of Trichotillomania Learning Center in Santa Cruz, California) used to tell me many times. It was evident in her own life, and it has been a phrase I remember often in day to day living.

It helps me very much to process, or work through, circumstances I am experiencing by either writing it down or talking to someone else. If I do this, I will most likely be able to identify the problem and work on changing it by learning what the real issue is behind it. The answer might not come immediately, but by bringing the real issue out, the answer does come. Trust your process. For me, the answer always came when I was ready for it.

My first real attempt at journal writing still makes me laugh when I think about it. I was venturing off on a new journey to "find myself," disturbed with the awareness that I really had no idea who I was. My empty white journal was in my hand as I went trekking up a sand dune along the coast in Davenport, California, to visit the sea lions. I planned to read a little of some recovery book and write whatever I discovered. I really did expect to process something that day, for I knew I was at a crossroads. I was desperate to find out who I really was. I had been in deep pain inside, recognizing that I really had no point of reference.

I remember walking up to the sea lions and being daring enough to step out of my frame of comfort by crossing over the ropes that were there to keep people on the correct path. I was rebelling, in a sense. I wanted to direct my own steps. Quietly I moved outside the ropes behind a tree and sat near some rocks a few feet from the water. I could see several sea lions to the left and right of me. I felt very comfortable and enjoyed the sound of the water and the seals. I began to write.

I remember being so terrified of what I'd find through the "door." I began to write something to the effect of, "Why am I so afraid to find out who stands on the other side of that door? I know it'll be me. Why would I actually have a feeling of terror?" I believe that as I wrote I began to feel a love, a yearning to know that person, me! I was opening myself up to her, inviting her in, not rejecting her as so many had. It was the beginning of a wonderful journey for which I will be grateful the rest of my life.

JOURNAL ENTRIES

These journal entries were written over a period of a few years. I wrote them as if I were writing to myself and to others, feeling that someday I might write a book and would want to include them in this type of chapter. So here is a look into my mind's process, to encourage you that if I can do it, you can too! I tried to choose excerpts that cover different stages of my recovery. Journal writing helps us identify our feelings and emotions. There is power in the pen. I encourage you to try it. Once again, if this overwhelms you, maybe you could begin by using a tape recorder.

October 3, 1994

> I'm feeling very angry and I realize that anger is a big prompter of my pulling. I don't know how to deal with anger. Lately I have had such a raging reaction to my kids when they act their ages. I don't know how to deal with my own frustrations. I am a person with very high expectations; more accurately, perfectionism. Sometimes I wonder how much of this came from my upbringing.

This entry let me state my feelings, which led to a revelation of the connection to my upbringing. From this came a "reparenting" in my life and a healing from the devastating repercussions of perfectionism.

(No date)

After pulling, sometimes I feel more okay about it than other times. What that tells me is that it's determined by my emotion.

When I realized that, I began to learn to stop and identify my emotions and redirect or reparent those negative feelings. I realized that if some days I can be okay, then maybe I can always feel okay!

(No date)

I have a lot of control issues. When I can't control my circumstances, I think I resort to something I can control, such as pulling.

This entry helped me look at my need for a sense of control. I think there are reasons for everything. If we can get in touch with the real cause, then we can have an appropriate response to how we handle a situation instead of striking out at others, hurting them, or doing inappropriate things.

(No date)

I am noticing that when I'm emotionally tired my brain just kind of shuts down and clicks off. It seems to take a lot of work to focus. So my assumption is that when I'm too tired to deal with stuff but I have a nervous energy, it is a dangerous

and powerful combination. Pulling fits right into
that niche; the combination of nervous energy
and wanting to vegetate, wanting to shut down.

From this entry I became aware that I needed to
change some of my living habits: earlier bedtimes and
no caffeine past 6 p.m., for example.

(No date)

One thing I'm noticing is that there are some
areas in my life I'm not happy about: my
parenting, lack of patience, lack of organizing,
and my attitude at times. I am realizing that I
need to make the effort to improve myself,
getting the help or instruction I need instead of
sitting back and not liking myself. I don't want
anything negative to dominate my life. I think I
have choices and it'll take a lot of courage to face
my inadequacies and dysfunctions, to go and do
the work to get better. I think that is crucial in
laying the groundwork so I can stop pulling. It
takes a lot of work. What is encouraging is that I
know that life will get better as I begin these steps.
I will get healthier emotionally.

206

(No date)

I want to learn to balance how much power I give away to people. I believe in being courteous and everything, but I've always tended to forsake myself to please someone else, in fear of them not liking me. For example, one night a while ago my daughter Alyson's coach was angry with me for not bringing her to practice. I was going through a shame attack around it and knew I didn't need to be reacting in that way. I owed nothing to this person. If he wanted to be angry, I needed to be able to let him feel his own feelings and not carry it for him. I know I can only do my best and that's that. I will never please everyone. I shouldn't overdramatize it or inflate it in my head, like it's a major big deal, when it really isn't. I called the instructor right away so I could get it out of my head. I didn't want to be thinking about it all day and obsessing over it. He said, "No big deal." Whether or not that was really true wasn't my problem. If he wanted to kick Alyson off of the team, then so be it.

The bottom line is that I just need to learn to look appropriately at situations. When I distort them it's spiritually and physically unhealthy, and I pull around those kinds of things.

One time when I was pulling all of my eyelashes out, I tried to convince myself to stop. I told myself, "Cheryn, a wedding is coming up and you want to have your eyelashes and eyebrows for the wedding." I was going to be around my family and sometimes it helps to get my head out of the situation when I look into the future. I'm still not always able to stop by saying, "Tomorrow I won't have eyelashes if I keep on pulling." It hasn't always worked for me, but I think that these are helpful ways to retrain the brain to think. I have heard other people say this, too. If there is some event coming up, I'm better able to leave my eyebrows or eyelashes in. It seems like the day after, though, they often come out anyway. I've heard a lot of people say that when they set a goal, they are better able to keep from pulling. When they don't set a goal, they have nothing to shoot for and they give in to the urge. I think that pretty well describes me, too.

(No date)

I ate almost half a big bag of potato chips, a Milky Way candy bar, and two Hostess cupcakes. That hasn't been my norm, and I don't know why. That's what I'm tired of, that's what I don't like.

(No date)

Lately I've been having memories of a few incidents of my childhood where my behavior was very inappropriate, due to my inability to understand and handle my feelings. For example, once my friend Cindy came over to stay the weekend and we were getting a little tired of each other. Instead of managing my feelings, I hid from her out by my mom's car in the driveway. For an hour or two my mom and Cindy called my name. I wouldn't come out until Cindy finally went home. I didn't know how to ask her to just go home. At least I could have asked my mom to nonchalantly ask her to leave. Why didn't I possess any skills? I just didn't seem to have any understanding, and I feel it goes deeper than just being immature.

March 5, 1990

Today I am beginning a journal again. I've been reaching out in a new way to others. I hope what happened to me last night was a spiritual breakthrough—through the wall of perfectionism and my fear of failure. I felt intense emotional sadness which I expressed through crying. It seemed to ease as I gave it up. I know when I am more capable I'll press harder into my school work, but just going to school and being a single parent has taken its toll and pushed me plenty.

When I felt overwhelmed and insecure, these last four days, I clung to Mike. Why do I do that? I felt so scared because my new experience of taking time off from myself really shook my foundation. I think I cling to those I feel are more planted and strong and able to help me, to carry me.

Is that why I don't know how to cling to myself instead of others?

June 13, 1990

I notice that I become obsessed with pulling out my hair when I'm lacking sleep but too tired to sleep. I'll have iced tea late at night and feel overwhelmed about stuff, especially if I have been pulling in previous days. Over the last three days I pulled out much of my pubic hair. I felt so terrible and went into a type of depression. I felt shame, like I had just torn out my femininity. I felt like I had lost ground. My identity's affirmation switched from positive to negative. I was doing really well a few days ago, reading my CoDa book, feeling so whole—even verbalizing how I felt like a whole woman. (Let me stress what a big statement that was, for I'd never felt that before.)

So here is the picture: three days ago I'm feeling like a completely whole woman, and now I've lost my identity for a day. Lost the vision of my wholeness. I refocused my eyes on my feminine appearance to define whether or not I was a woman. Where are my internal boundaries?

The state of mind I go into when I'm pulling is such a grievance for me in my life because I now see it a deeper, clearer way. The place I've hidden in for so long is a place I no longer want to be.

(No date)

Last night I drank two glasses of iced tea and went to bed around 12:30 p.m. Then I stressed for 2 1/2 hours pulling on the few eyebrows I have and eliminating any stubs of eyelashes. I felt under "its" power to pull but I did try to work some recovery steps into the busyness of my chaotic mind. "Okay Cheryn, breathe, meditate," lasts an average of three to five seconds when I'm in this state. Then I'm off again in three different directions. (*Author's note: I now believe*

Attention Deficit Disorder, ADD, was the cause of much of that, if not all.) I thought, "Why am I unable to be 'here?'" and then I felt myself, with a glimpse of awareness, return to the present. I recognized feelings of guilt; guilt which covered so many issues, so many areas of my life. I realized partially why my mind races. I feel overwhelmed, not okay about being imperfect, so I have learned to not be "here" and spin out emotionally.

I've had walls of protection up for so long, keeping out pain. The pain of the unknown and of pain itself. So much seemed to bring me pain that I hid pretty often. I'd pull my eyelashes if anyone hurt my feelings, which most often was daily. Once in a while a breath of relief would come, and for a period of time I would not feel compelled to pull.

March 6, 1995

Today was a tough day. I pulled my eyelashes out last night and my left eyelid was swollen noticeably, adding insult to injury. I was more depressed than I had been in a long time. In church yesterday the passage talked about was our "significance" to God. These were the questions I asked myself today to try to put things in perspective:

"Am I lesser than anyone else? No! Why do I put so much emphasis on eyelashes? They are only a physical part of my being." This helped me to recognize my true significance. I am now very aware of how society teaches that you have to be a "star" (wealthy, beautiful, thin, etc.) to be significant. I've always believed that, too, since I was a child, but now I reject this concept completely. I know I was not alone in this way of thinking. What a shame. There is so much pain in that concept of reality. It amazes me how this philosophy sticks like super glue to the pores of our self-esteem. Occasionally, it still rears its ugly head, though I do notice that it is less and less often. I can see that as lies are replaced with truth, truth does overcome.

September 20, 1994

I just finished pulling. "Finished" is said with hope attached to it.

September 27, 1994

I just got out of bed to come write because once again after a deep silent cry over pulling, I was struck with how familiar my pain was. It was like the pain I had when I was twelve years old.

January 12, 1993

I occupy my mind continually in a way that keeps me busy and out of the present.

November 4, 1992

My body's energy is very compulsively focused. It goes wherever my mind does not. When I have a project, I can't feel settled again until it's finished completely. I recognize no balance.

January 21, 1995

I believe my pulling episodes reflect my present life's conditions. I've been emotionally isolating myself and feeling no ability to stop. I'm becoming aware of how this is more a reflection of me and am beginning to look at it. I don't pull anymore for just any occasion. That behavior has ceased due to my awareness work. I can stop more easily if I remember to examine the situation in my life during that time. That pretty much reverses the binge quickly. This is the hard part. Discipline has never been one of my strong points. To me it's like exercising even when I don't want to, knowing that there is a great reward after I'm done. It's also like eating the right thing instead of carelessly eating harmful trigger foods. They give sweetness in the mouth but bitterness in my stomach, like the way chocolate causes jitters, anxiousness, sleeplessness, weight gain, and sugar cravings.

I believe if I can make the first choice with love, I'll make the right choice. First I have to learn to love.

(No date)

I don't feel very loved right now from Michael, and I know it's all about me. His feelings haven't changed, mine have (about myself). This is the same stuff I dealt with in my youth. I always felt unloved and insecure, to the worst degree. I loathed myself. I felt I was worth nothing. I rejected anyone's love. I felt, "How could anyone love me?" I always seem to be needing reassurance.

August 10, 1994

Looking at my eyes triggers my pulling. So I tell myself, "Don't look!" Why is this step taking so long for me to get? How long will it be before I can look and not pull? Why can't I remember the pain of how I feel after each pulling episode is over? If I could feel, then I'd stop, right?

If I want to be whole, I need to heal. It is my time. It is our time. I believe we plant seeds throughout our youth, and who we are as adults is the product of those seeds' growth. No matter how we look, we are all so much more beautiful on the inside than on the outside. Sadly, we are not in a society that possesses this viewpoint. We need to stand up for ourselves and claim what is rightfully ours. We were all created with an inner beauty. Some decide to look for it, others don't.

I have never seen someone with outward beauty to be greater than a person who has found their inner beauty. I have felt a deep connection with every person who I have met with Trich. It seems that there is a beauty we all possess. We have learned lessons from not basing our identities on our outside appearance. Sure, we might start out feeling negative toward our physical appearance, but I believe because of this we learn to look a little bit deeper. I know I am not alone in expressing this. I have gone to four annual retreats of the Trichotillomania Learning Center in Santa Cruz, California, and have gathered with nearly one hundred people each time. I am amazed at the similarities and the special bond we share. I am truly grateful to be a part of our "club." We are all blessed, and we can only discover this when we become overcomers of this condition.

Remember to embrace your life experiences and accept them. You wouldn't be who you are today.

The following are a few poems I selected that are close to my heart. I wanted to share this private part of myself with you.

Dear God,

Please plant me solidly on this earth.

Give me roots that go deep.

Make me grow tall and wide with limbs that bear fruit that nourishes myself and others.

Let my growth be empowered by Your Spirit, that all my fruit will not die,

But will become seed that will reproduce and multiply.

Help me understand myself and life and know you deeply.

© 1995 Cheryn Salazar

 It used to be my heart would cry
But now it's made to sing.
I truly claim that sorrows past
Have brought me depths of joy at last.
Though painful as the road has been,
I would choose to travel this road again
For it has taught me who I am
And that my life does have a plan.
The road I traveled was lonely and long,
And certainly with much cost,
But what and who I've found I am
Has shown me no experience was lost.
Now my heart has a new song
For my worth is not found in my hair.
It takes great courage to look elsewhere,
To look elsewhere than there.

© 1995 Cheryn Salazar

BROKEN DREAMS

As children bring their broken toys
With tears for us to mend,
I brought my broken dreams to God
Because He was my friend.
But then, instead of leaving Him
In peace to work alone,
I hung around and tried to help
With ways that were my own.
At last, I snatched them back and cried,
"How can you be so slow?"
"My child," he said,
"What could I do?"
"You never did let go."

(Author unknown.)

TRICHOTILLOMANIA LEARNING CENTER (TLC)

The Trichotillomania Learning Center, Inc. (TLC) is a national nonprofit organization supported by memberships. It was established in 1991 by a sufferer of the condition. TLC provides information, support, and referral resources to all who inquire about the experience and treatment of compulsive hair pulling.

Although there have been no epidemiological studies to identify the actual number of people with this condition yet, it is estimated that in the United States alone there are probably between six and eight million sufferers of Trichotillomania.

The purpose of establishing TLC was to assist in the development of treatment options for those suffering from compulsive hair pulling and other related behaviors. Their goal is to insure that this information is accessible to those in need, through them or from other resources.

With the growing need for professionals specializing in this field, TLC is also committed to providing the most up-to-date information available on diagnosis and treatment, along with continuing to work toward public awareness and education to fulfill these goals. TLC has a comprehensive information package on Trichotillomania that can be ordered by contacting them. Their address is TLC, 1215 Mission St., Santa Cruz, CA 95060. (Reprinted with TLC approval.)

TLC'S ANNUAL RETREAT

Each year, TLC holds an annual retreat allowing people to come together in a safe and private environment for a few days of rest, information and recovery. This provides a chance to step outside the veil of secrecy, a chance to play and make new friends, and continues to aid in the development of a loving national network of support.

❧ 13 ❧

CONCLUSION

Conclusion

I can say that regardless of whether I continue to pull or not, a new love for myself has developed over the years. It has taken time, much work and patience (an attribute I reach for on a daily basis). Life is good. If we can overcome and grow beyond our circumstances, then we can experience it in the manner we were intended.

I have written this book over a period of several years. Many of my reflections stemmed from different stages of my pulling. As I finish writing this book my urges to pull are minimal, and my Trich is under management. I credit my success on the things I have written about in this book. I wrote this book as I've lived it. I know Trich will always be a part of my psyche, but I no longer have to be a slave to it.

The following is a true story about a mule who fell in a well sixty feet deep. The owner of the mule did not want to shoot her, knowing her fate, so he tried burying her with truckloads of dirt. As he would drop dirt on her, the mule would shake off the dirt and stomp on the fallen dirt, packing it down. She would do this each time the soil fell upon her back. After three loads of dirt, the owner saw what was happening. He kept dumping soil until the mule was able to ascend out of the well on her own.

I love this story because I believe it is a picture of my experience. It can be a picture of your experience, as well. The pain that trichotillomania often causes can either destroy us emotionally and physically, or be a prompter or a stepping stone to help us look deeper into our being.

My road to recovery and experience of healing and restoration has been incredible and deeply spiritual. I always have held a belief in God as a creator, but never felt He was a personal God who could have an intimate relationship with His creations. I also believed He had abandoned me over the years regarding my Trichotillomania. Today I know that He was answering my prayers, just in a different way. I am grateful, because of the growth and lessons I've learned in my life, that He didn't remove my Trich when I asked Him. I always believed that trials and suffering were bad, but today I understand that during these times my character grows and I develop emotionally. I would not be who I am today if I had not experienced Trichotillomania.

Today, I also know Him. I experience a personal relationship with my creator, which began when I asked Jesus Christ to forgive me of my sins. He then revealed Himself to me and lives in me and through me with His Holy Spirit. (I have spoken of my spiritual beliefs and of God in my book, knowing that some might be offended, but this book is all about my life and experiences. To leave God out of them now would be an inaccuracy.) His strength truly is my strength. His love has healed my deepest hurts. I wouldn't say it if it weren't true, for being a Christian isn't exactly a very popular position in our world today. Many people have shamed the name of Christianity.

Even if you don't share my beliefs, I hope you can glean something for yourself from this book. It was written with love, not preachiness, in mind. I personally dislike someone who is preachy; but someone who cares about me, who knows my pain and offers acceptance and understanding can share their beliefs and helpful ideas without making me uncomfortable. I hope you feel the same way.

I hope you will hear my heart and know that my beliefs are so integrated into my life and my being that this book could not have been written without including the spiritual part of me. My prayer is that some part of this book will have helped you in some way, hopefully many ways, to find your own precious worth.

This is, to me, the most important message I could ever give. Because I care, I am going to end this book with my beliefs.

I believe in the God of the Bible, who is loving, forgiving and intimately knows each of us. He even knows how many hairs are on our head (Matthew 10:30), or aren't! I believe in the Bible as the word of God and that Jesus Christ is God incarnate (John 1:1-13), and that Jesus was crucified and resurrected and is living today. I have experienced His Holy Spirit in my life for many years now, just as He promised in Acts 2 of the New Testament. It has been that way since the day I sought Him from the depths of my being, asking Him to reveal Himself if He were real.

This book is about me. I have written it with love and compassion to you, my friend. I've probably never met you, but I know you—a very secret part of you. I am grateful that now you know me, too. We are not alone anymore.

SUGGESTED READING
AUDIO/VISUAL AIDS
&
PRODUCTS

Suggested Reading, Visual Aids, Products and Other Resources

Books:

Whats Happening to My Child: A Guide for Parents of Hair Pullers
By Cheryn Salazar
This is a helpful, easy to understand book for parents of kids with Trich. Best of all, it's written by a woman who has struggled with the issue herself, as well as raised two children with the same disorder. The book's filled with hope and hints to overcoming despair. By offering loving and compassionate recognition of both the parents needs, and the needs of the child who is pulling. Cheryn's message is one of support, honest and deep commitment to the recovery process of a healthy family.
Available through Cheryn.com, Trich.org, and Amazon.com

The Hair Pulling "Habit" and You
By R. Golomb and S. Vavrichek
This workbook for young Trichotillomania sufferers is written in plain common-sense language and allows each user to tailor the program to his or her own needs. The information is highly accessible to children, and is based upon the latest understandings of Trichotillomania. Recommended to younger people, parents, and therapists as well.

For more information go to
www.hairpullinghabit.com
Available through TLC's Book and Video Order
Form @ trich.org as well as Amazon.com
*The Hair Pulling Problem: A Complete guide to
Trichotillomania*
By Fred Penzel, Ph.D.

This book includes all the information a patient or
relative would need to understand this illness and
cope with it. Dr. Penzel provides a detailed
discussion of the causes and he reviews all the
treatment options, with particular emphasis upon
cognitive and behavioral therapies, as well as the
most effective medications and their side effects.
He shows patients how to design a self-help
program and gain control over their compulsive
behaviors, how to prevent relapse, describes
Trichotillomania and its treatment in children, and
suggest coping strategies for families at home and
in public situations.
Available through TLC's Book and Video Order
Form @Trich.org as well as Amazon.com

*Help for Hair Pullers: Understanding and Coping
with Trichotillomania*
By Nancy J. Keuthen, Ph.D., Dan J. Stein, M.D.,
and Gary A. Christenson, M.D.

This book reviews the latest treatment options and
offers effective cognitive-behavioral techniques for

controlling this disorder. For more information go to www.trichhelp.com

Available through TLC's Book and Video Order Form @ Trich.org as well as Amazon.com

Trichotillomania
By Dan J. Stein M.B., Gary Christenson M.D., and Eric Hollander, M.D. (editors)

This book has been written from a clinical and a research perspective by psychiatrists, psychologists, and researchers and covers issues such as assessment, childhood Trichotillomania, the role of hypnotherapy and the relationship between Trichotillomania and OCD. The use of medication, the place of a psychodynamic perspective and the value of behavioral interventions are also thoroughly discussed. Recommended for treatment providers, and people studying Trichotillomania.

Available through Amazon.com

Your Best Life Now, 7 Steps to Living At Your Full Potential

By Joel Osteen
A marvelous book about reaching the potential you were born to embrace. Available at bookstores nationwide and on Amazon.com
The following books are by Henry Cloud & John Townsend:
Boundaries
Boundaries with Kids
Boundaries in Marriage
Raising Great Kids
Raising Great Kids for Parents of Preschoolers
Raising Great Kids for Parents of Teenagers
How People Grow
Changes That Heal
Safe People
The Mom Factor
Make Room For Daddy

The Following Books are by Dr. James Dobson:
Parents' Answer Book: A Comprehensive Resource From America's Most Respected Parenting Expert
Preparing for Adolescence
The New Hide or Seek
The New Strong-Willed Child
The New Dare to Discipline
Parenting Isn't for Cowards
Bringing Up Boys
Night Light for Parents
Certain Peace in Uncertain Times
Dr. Dobson: Turning Hearts Toward Home
Love Must Be Tough: New Hope for Marriages

in Crisis
Complete Marriage and Family Home
  Reference Guide
Straight Talk to Men
TLC Email News List:
Sign up today! This is a free and easy way for you to stay up to date with TLC and Trichotillomania. When you sign up for this email list, you will receive a message anytime there is news from TLC.

TLC will send you email about:
Scientific research reports
Research studies you can participate in
Conferences, retreats
Local networking events
Media appearances
New resources, books, organizations, and
  products
TLC Volunteer projects
How you can help TLC

TRICHOTILLOMANIA LEARNING CENTER
303 Potrero St. #51, Santa Cruz, CA 95060
(831) 457-1004 / fax: (831) 426-4383
www.trich.org

Videos:

"Our Personal Stories – The Truth of Trichotillomania"

TLC has produced a documentary video on the experience of Trichotillomania called "Our Personal Stories – The Truth of Trichotillomania." This video expresses some of the life situations and areas of personal grief and recovery experienced by the eight women on the tape. For anyone seeking personal insight into this disorder, this tape is highly useful.

For more information for purchasing this video go to www.trich.org

"Bad Hair Life" – A documentary film by Jennifer Raikes

This vivid one-hour documentary explores the often deeply secretive disorder, Trichotillomania, or compulsive hair-pulling. The idea for this film grew out of the personal experience of Jennifer Raikes, a producer at Middlemarch Films, who has had Trichotillomania for over 20 years. Five years in the making, the documentary is the first in depth portrayal of this complex disorder and the profound impact it has on the lives of those struggling with it.

The documentary presents intimate portraits of adults and children at different stages of coping with hair-pulling. Using art, photography and interviews, *Bad Hair Life* examines the importance of hair to our identities and the cultural forces that make this disorder feel shameful.

The director shares her own history with hair-pulling, starting when she was nine and idly pulled out her first eyelash, through years of embarrassment and hiding, to her present quest to understand this mysterious behavior. Expert researchers and clinicians discuss the disorder's causes and treatment. But the film's greatest power is in its intensely honest, first-hand accounts of life with Trichotillomania. For more information for purchasing this video go to www.trich.org

Products Specifically Developed for Those Who've Experienced Hair Loss

Cheryn International is a company that grew out of Cheryn Salazar's personal experience with Trichotillomania. She developed a line of truly natural-looking false eyelashes and various makeup products to subtly enhance the beauty of those who have experienced various types of hair loss. Cheryn's desire is to provide a feeling of normalcy and beauty.

For further information, or to contact Cheryn Salazar about speaking engagements, please write or call:

Cheryn Salazar
15227 Medella Circle
Rancho Murieta, CA 95683
(916) 804-1337
CherynS@Cheryn.com